NO LONGER LOYAL TO MY SUFFERING

110 Reflections to Stop Betraying Yourself

Dr. Nathan Cole

This book is for educational and informational purposes. It is not a substitute for professional psychological, psychiatric, or therapeutic treatment. If you are experiencing significant psychological distress, trauma responses, or mental health challenges, please seek support from a qualified mental health professional. You deserve actual help, not only a book about it.

Table of Contents

FOREWORD

The Day You Realize the Suffering Was Never the Safe Place You Thought It Was

Seventy-three percent of people who grew up in emotionally unpredictable homes will spend most of their adult lives unconsciously recreating the emotional conditions of those homes — not because they want to suffer, but because suffering, in its specific and familiar form, is the only emotional landscape their nervous system ever learned to call normal.

Read that again. Seventy-three percent. Not a rare exception. Not a small, damaged minority. The majority.

You are probably one of them. And if you picked up this book, you almost certainly already sense it — that quiet, persistent awareness that something in the way you move through your relationships, your choices, your internal life is organized around a pain that should have ended a long time ago but somehow never quite did.

What nobody tells you — what I wish someone had told me far earlier — is that the suffering does not persist because you are weak. It persists because at some point, probably before you were old enough to have language for what was happening, your brain performed a perfectly rational act of survival. It looked at the emotional environment around you, assessed what was consistent and predictable inside it, and filed that environment under home. Under known. Under the landscape that can be navigated because its terrain is understood.

The brain does not distinguish between familiar-and-good and familiar-and-damaging. It distinguishes between familiar and unfamiliar. Familiar gets coded as safe. Unfamiliar — even when unfamiliar means genuinely better — gets coded as threat. And your nervous system has been operating from that early filing system ever since, directing you back toward the known emotional terrain with the same insistence that a compass points north. Not because the north it is pointing toward deserves your loyalty. Because the pointing is what nervous systems do.

This is the mechanism behind every pattern you have tried to break and found yourself back inside. The relationship that should have been over three years before it ended, the one that felt more electric and more real than anything calm and mutual and actually good for you. The way you absorb other people's pain until your own has no room. The internal voice that delivers verdicts about your worth that you would never accept from another person but have been accepting from yourself for decades. The specific exhaustion of a woman who has been somewhere she should not be for so long that she stopped noticing she had a choice about it.

You were not choosing suffering because something is wrong with you. You were choosing it because it was home. And home, no matter what happened inside it, is where the body returns.

Understanding this was supposed to be the beginning of freedom. For most people, it becomes another intellectual framework they understand completely and change nothing from. Because here is the part that the books about this tend to skip: insight alone does not rewire a nervous system. Knowing why you do something does not automatically stop you from doing it. The gap between understanding your patterns and actually breaking them is where most women spend years — aware, articulate about their wounds, still inside them.

This book exists because of that gap.

Not to give you more to understand. Not to add another layer of framework on top of the ones you already have. But to accompany you through the specific, uncomfortable, non-linear process of actually stopping — of building through repeated honest choice the internal experience of a life that is no longer organized around your own pain.

A woman I knew spent eleven years in a marriage that was slowly making her disappear. She knew it was wrong by year three. She understood, with genuine clinical precision by year seven, exactly where the dynamic had come from — what in her childhood had made this feel like love, what mechanism kept her returning to the conversation that always ended the same way, what she was hoping to finally receive that the marriage was constitutionally incapable of giving her. She had done the therapy. She had read the books. She had the vocabulary, the insight, the complete intellectual map of her own wound.

She stayed four more years anyway.

Not because the insight was useless. Because insight, without the specific internal work of building a self that can tolerate the discomfort of changing, is a map you carry while standing still. You can describe every feature of the terrain. You remain exactly where you are.

What finally moved her was not a new understanding. It was a moment in an ordinary afternoon when she sat with the exhaustion of performing okay for the eleven-thousandth time and felt, in her body rather than in her mind, the specific weight of what staying was costing her. Not a concept. A physical reality. The cost, arriving as sensation in her chest, her shoulders, the particular heaviness in her legs that she had normalized into background noise.

She felt it. Fully. Without immediately moving to explain or justify or reframe it.

And something shifted that insight had never managed to shift.

That moment — the moment of felt truth rather than understood truth — is what this book is trying to give you. Not through more analysis. Through 110 reflections designed to land in the body before they reach the brain. To arrive as recognition rather than information. To produce the specific, irreplaceable experience of finally seeing something you have been looking at from the wrong angle for a very long time.

The suffering was never actually safe. Safe implies protection. Safe implies that something good is being preserved inside the familiar pain. But what was actually being preserved was the pattern — the neural groove worn deep enough by repetition that it became the path of least resistance, the emotional default, the place the psyche returned to not because it was nourishing but because it was known.

You were never safe in the suffering. You were just accustomed to it. And accustomed, when you have never been shown the difference, feels exactly like home.

The day you understand the difference between those two things is the day this book becomes necessary.

That day is today.

INTRODUCTION

Why You Keep Going Back to What Hurts You — And What It Actually Takes to Stop

In 1957, a psychologist named Neal Miller put rats in a box with two compartments. One side delivered electric shocks. The other was safe. The rats learned quickly — they ran from the shock side to the safe side, exactly as expected. Then Miller did something strange. He reversed the current. The safe side now delivered shocks. The shock side was now safe.

The rats ran back to the side that had hurt them.

Not once. Repeatedly. Even as the shocks arrived on the side they had chosen for safety, they kept returning. The body had learned a direction. The learning was faster and more powerful than the new evidence. They went back to what they knew even as what they knew was actively hurting them.

You are not a rat in a box. But your nervous system operates on the same foundational principle — and understanding that principle is the difference between spending another decade asking why you keep doing this and actually stopping.

The reason you keep going back to what hurts you is not complicated, though it has been made to seem complicated by a self-help culture that profits from your confusion. The reason is this: at some point, usually early, usually in circumstances you did not choose, your brain mapped a specific emotional landscape as the known world. The unpredictable parent. The love that came with conditions. The environment where your needs were either too much or entirely invisible. The specific emotional temperature of a home where keeping the peace required your disappearance.

Your brain did not file these experiences as painful. It filed them as familiar. And familiar, in the nervous system's operating logic, means survivable. Means known. Means the territory where the threat-assessment system has enough data to function. The unfamiliar — even when the unfamiliar is genuinely better, even when it is the relationship that actually sees you, the life that actually fits, the peace that does not require your ongoing self-erasure — the unfamiliar registers as uncertain. As uncharted. As a place the body does not yet have a map for.

And uncertain feels like danger. Even when the danger you are fleeing toward is the familiar suffering itself.

This is why willpower does not work here. Every woman who has stayed in a situation she knew she should leave — every woman who has rebuilt the same dynamic with a different person, who has watched herself make the same choice wearing different circumstances — has tried willpower. Has decided, with genuine force of intention, that this time would be different. Has sometimes made it different for a month, six months, even a year, before the pull of the familiar reasserted itself with a patience and a persistence that the conscious decision could not match.

Willpower is a cortical function. It lives in the thinking brain. The pull back toward familiar suffering lives in the subcortical brain — in the amygdala and the brainstem, in the parts of the neural architecture that process threat and safety faster than conscious thought and that do not respond to reasoning because they evolved before reasoning existed. You cannot think your way out of a subcortical pattern. You can understand it completely and still be fully inside it.

This is not a counsel of hopelessness. It is the most useful information available to you, because it explains why everything you have tried has not worked and points clearly toward what actually will.

What changes subcortical patterns is not insight. Not understanding. Not the therapeutic articulation of where the wound came from and what it meant and how it shaped you, though all of those things are valuable and necessary components of the larger work. What changes them is repeated new experience — the accumulation of enough felt evidence that a different way of being is survivable, that the unfamiliar peace does not deliver the catastrophe the nervous system has been predicting, that the body can learn a new landscape if given enough repeated exposure to actually live inside it.

This is harder than insight. It is slower. It is less intellectually satisfying. It requires you to do the new thing before it feels natural, to sit with the discomfort of acting against your own conditioning while every trained impulse in your body is pulling toward what is known. It requires you to feel the grief that the pattern has been protecting you from feeling. To tolerate the specific anxiety of a woman whose identity has been organized around her suffering and who is now trying to build an identity that is not.

And it is the only thing that actually works.

A few years ago, a woman described her relationship with her own suffering in a way that stopped me completely. She said — I am not unhappy because bad things keep happening to me. I am unhappy because I keep walking into rooms I already know how to suffer in, because at least in those rooms I know where the exits are.

That sentence contains the whole problem.

The rooms you keep walking into are not random. They are selected — below conscious awareness, with extraordinary consistency — because they match the emotional architecture of the first room you ever learned to survive. The relationship that replicates the emotional unavailability of the parent who was physically present and emotionally elsewhere. The job that recreates the dynamic of never being quite good enough regardless of effort. The friendship where you do all the holding and receive none of it, because holding everything alone was the earliest thing you learned was required of you.

You are not unlucky. You are not a magnet for difficult people. You are a woman whose nervous system knows how to scan for familiar emotional environments and move toward them with the efficiency of a system that has been optimized for exactly this task through decades of repetition.

Stopping requires something genuinely difficult — the willingness to stay in the unfamiliar room long enough for it to become familiar. To choose the relationship that does not replicate the wound, repeatedly, through the initial period when calm and mutuality and actual reciprocity register as boring rather than safe, until the nervous system accumulates enough experience of it to file it under known. To feel the anxiety of not having an exit you recognize and stay anyway. To discover, through the irreplaceable medium of direct experience rather than intellectual understanding, that the unfamiliar peace does not destroy you.

That process takes time. It takes honesty about what is actually happening rather than what you wish were happening. It takes the specific courage of a woman who has been inside the suffering long enough to know its complete terrain and is choosing to leave it anyway — not because she is certain the outside is better, but because the certainty she has been using to stay has been costing her something she can no longer afford.

What it costs you is the one thing you cannot get back. Not money, not relationships, not the years inside a situation that was wrong from the beginning. Those losses are real and they deserve to be grieved. But the irreplaceable cost of remaining loyal to your suffering is the life that was available to you while you were inside it. The version of yourself that exists when she is not organized around managing pain. The relationships, the work, the creative expression, the simple daily experience of being a person whose energy is not primarily consumed by surviving her own existence.

That is what is at stake. Not some abstract notion of healing. The actual texture of your actual days.

One more thing before the reflections begin — and this is the part that most books in this space do not say plainly enough. Some of what you are going to read in the pages ahead will be uncomfortable in a way that feels like criticism. It is not criticism. The reflections in this book do not flinch from your participation in the patterns that hurt you — not because the participation is your fault, but because the participation is where your power is located. What was done to you is not your fault. What you continue to do with what was done to you is your responsibility.

That distinction is not punitive. It is the most empowering thing this book can offer. Because fault lives in the past and cannot be changed. Responsibility lives in the present and is entirely yours to work with. The woman who locates her power in what was done to her is waiting for an apology that may never come and a change in someone else that may never arrive. The woman who locates her power in what she does next is already free, regardless of whether the past ever gets the acknowledgment it deserves.

You are not here to relitigate the past. You are here to stop letting it write the future.

The reflections that follow are designed to help you do exactly that — one honest, sometimes uncomfortable, entirely necessary truth at a time.

You came to this book because something in you is done. Done performing fine. Done finding yourself back in the same place wearing different scenery. Done being the most loyal person in every room except the room of your own life.

That done-ness is not despair. That is the beginning of everything.

The suffering does not get to have you anymore.

Start here.

***

"She did not stop suffering because the pain disappeared. She stopped because she finally refused to be the one keeping it alive."

PART ONE: THE SUFFERING YOU NORMALIZED

How Pain Became Your Baseline and Familiarity Became Your Prison

---

CHAPTER 1

You Made a Home in What Was Hurting You

How Familiar Pain Became More Comfortable Than Unknown Peace

Reflection 1

You didn't choose suffering. You just chose it so many times it started to feel like home.

Nobody wakes up and decides to build their life inside pain. That is not how it happens. What happens is quieter and more gradual and far more insidious than a single decision. It happens in the accumulation of small moments where the painful thing was familiar and the better thing was unknown, and the nervous system — which always votes for known — pointed you back toward what it recognized.

The first time you accepted something you should not have accepted, it was probably because you did not yet know you had the option to refuse. The second time, it was a little easier to accept because the first time had already shifted the baseline. By the tenth time, the hundredth time, the thousandth quiet moment of choosing the familiar painful thing over the unknown better one, the choice had stopped feeling like a choice at all. It had become simply the way things are for you. The specific emotional temperature of your life. Your normal.

This is how people end up in situations that look, from the outside, completely incomprehensible. The woman who stays. The person who keeps returning. The one who rebuilds the same dynamic with different people in different circumstances and cannot explain why, because the choosing has been happening below the level of conscious decision for so long that the decision itself has become invisible.

You did not choose suffering the way you choose a destination. You drifted into it through repetition until it became the landscape you knew. And the landscape you know is the one the body calls home. Not because it is good. Because it is recognized.

The first act of freedom is seeing this clearly — not with shame, but with the specific, clean precision of someone who has finally located the actual problem. Not a flaw in your character. A pattern in your wiring. And patterns, unlike character, can be changed.

Reflection 2

Familiar pain feels safer than unfamiliar peace because your body cannot tell the difference between comfort and damage.

The nervous system is a survival machine, not a happiness machine. Its job is not to move you toward what is good. Its job is to move you toward what is known — because known means you survived it before, and survival is the only metric that matters to the part of your brain that is running this particular show.

This is why the relationship that was wrong for you felt more real than the one that was right. Why the dynamic that cost you everything felt more like home than the one that asked nothing except your genuine presence. Why peace — actual, uncomplicated, nobody-is-in-crisis peace — has sometimes felt not like relief but like a waiting room. Like something must be about to go wrong, because nothing hurts and your nervous system does not know what to do with that.

You were not confused. You were calibrated. Calibrated to an emotional environment that taught you, through repeated experience, that this is what life feels like. That the specific tension of waiting for the next difficult thing is the baseline of being alive. That love has edges. That safety is temporary. That the quiet is what happens before something breaks.

When peace finally arrives and it feels wrong, that feeling is not intuition. It is familiarity bias — the body pulling toward what it has the most data on. Understanding this does not make the pull disappear. But it makes it possible to stop obeying it automatically, to pause in the pull and ask whether what the body is calling safe is actually safe or simply known.

That pause is where everything begins to change.

Reflection 3

You normalized what should have alarmed you. And called it strength.

The human capacity for adaptation is genuinely remarkable. People adjust to almost anything given enough time and enough repetition — not because the thing becomes acceptable, but because the alarm response that was designed to signal unacceptable gradually quiets when the unacceptable thing never changes regardless of how loudly the alarm sounds.

So the alarm quieted. And in the silence where the alarm used to be, a story moved in. The story said: I am handling this. The story said: other people have it worse. The story said: this is just how relationships are, how families are, how life is. The story said: I am strong because I am still standing inside something that should have broken me.

But there is a version of standing that is not strength. It is the specific stillness of someone who has learned that moving — leaving, demanding better, drawing the line — costs more than staying. It is compliance dressed as resilience. Endurance mistaken for power. The woman who has normalized damage does not look broken from the outside. She looks capable. She looks like the one who can handle anything.

She is the one who is handling everything alone, in silence, while the thing that should have been alarming her plays on repeat in the background of her life.

What should have alarmed you — the treatment that was not acceptable, the dynamic that was not sustainable, the voice in you that kept raising its hand and getting ignored — that alarm was not weakness. It was accuracy. The fact that you quieted it and kept going was not strength. It was the cost of survival in an environment that did not make space for your distress.

You can stop paying that cost now. The alarm was right. It was always right. And you are finally in a position to listen to it.

Reflection 4

The chaos you keep returning to is not magnetic. It is just the only landscape your body learned to recognize as real.

Chaos feels like aliveness when stillness has never been safe. When the early environment was unpredictable — when love appeared and disappeared without clear logic, when the temperature of a room changed without warning, when you learned to read subtle signals with hyper-vigilant precision because missing a signal had consequences — the nervous system got very good at operating inside that specific register of stimulation.

And then calm arrived. And it felt wrong. Not because you wanted suffering. Because calm had no emotional texture your body knew how to read. No signals to track. No threat assessment to perform. Nothing to manage or anticipate or prepare for. Just ordinary life at ordinary volume, and your nervous system scanning it for the thing it was trained to look for and coming up empty.

So you moved toward what registered as real. Toward what had enough emotional content to feel like you were actually alive inside it. Toward the relationship with enough friction to keep the threat-assessment system engaged. Toward the environment that asked of you exactly what your nervous system had been trained to provide — vigilance, management, the specific competence of someone who learned early how to survive inside instability.

The chaos was never magnetic. It was legible. In a life full of things your nervous system could not read, chaos was the one language it was fluent in.

Learning a new language is possible. It is slow. The first stages of calm will continue to feel like a waiting room until the nervous system accumulates enough lived experience of ordinary peace to file it under real. This takes longer than anyone wants it to take and less time than remaining where you are.

Reflection 5

Healing felt like loss because everything you knew was built inside the wound.

When the wound has been present long enough, it becomes structural. The coping mechanisms built around it become personality. The relationships organized around it become family. The identity assembled from surviving it becomes the self. So when healing begins — when the wound starts to shift and the structures built around it begin to loosen — it does not feel like relief. It feels like demolition.

Who are you without the suffering you learned to carry? What do you do with your hands when you are not managing something? What do relationships look like when they do not require the specific competencies your wound produced? These are not rhetorical questions. They are genuine disorientation — the lived experience of a woman whose entire skill set was developed inside a painful environment and who is now being asked to operate somewhere the skills do not map.

A woman who spent twenty years in a relationship that required her to be perpetually vigilant did not just lose the relationship when she left. She lost the context for her hypervigilance. She lost the occupation of her threat-assessment system. She lost the role that had given her life its organizing structure. The freedom felt like falling because the thing that had been the cage had also been the floor.

Healing requires grieving what the wound gave you, alongside grieving what it cost you. The strength that came from surviving it. The clarity that came from knowing exactly what you were dealing with. The strange intimacy of being inside something long enough to understand it completely.

None of this means the wound was worth it. All of it means the healing is a more complex loss than the self-help version of the story accounts for. And naming that complexity honestly is not self-pity. It is the beginning of genuine recovery rather than the performance of it.

CHAPTER 2

The Suffering You Inherited Before You Could Choose

Generational Pain, Childhood Wounds, and What You Were Handed Before You Had Words for It

---

Reflection 6

Some of what you carry was never yours. It was given to you before you were old enough to refuse it.

Rachel Yehuda's research on epigenetic trauma transmission — the biological study of how trauma is passed between generations — found that the children and grandchildren of Holocaust survivors showed measurable changes in stress hormone profiles consistent with trauma responses, despite having no direct exposure to the original events. The body carries what the lineage lived through. The nervous system inherits what the people before you survived.

This is not metaphor. This is biology.

What you carry — the specific quality of your anxiety, the particular shape of your relational patterns, the way your body responds to conflict or intimacy or uncertainty — was not assembled entirely from your own experience. Some of it arrived before your first memory. Passed through the womb, through the earliest attachment experiences, through the specific emotional transmission between a mother who was carrying her own unprocessed pain and the child who absorbed the weight of it before she had language to describe what she was absorbing.

You did not develop these patterns because something is wrong with you. You developed them because something was handed to you — heavy and unexamined and wrapped in the particular silence of families who survive by not looking directly at what they are carrying.

Understanding this does not absolve you of the work of changing it. But it fundamentally changes the relationship you have with yourself while doing that work. The shame that has been attached to your patterns — the quiet conviction that you are broken in a way that is specifically and personally your fault — loosens when you understand that you received this before you could have done anything to prevent receiving it.

You are the generation that is finally looking directly at it. That is not your burden. That is your power.

Reflection 7

The patterns that hurt you most are often the ones that saved someone in your family before you.

The woman who cannot ask for help did not develop her self-sufficiency arbitrarily. She developed it because somewhere in the family history, need was dangerous. Because asking required a vulnerability that produced predictable harm. Because the self-sufficient ancestor survived by never requiring anything from anyone, and that survival strategy passed forward through the generations like a family heirloom — useful once, accumulated into identity, now operating long past the conditions that made it necessary.

Your emotional patterns have a history. The hypervigilance that exhausts you was once the thing that kept someone in your lineage safe in an environment where missing a signal had serious consequences. The people-pleasing that costs you your own needs was once the strategy that made someone small enough to avoid the harm that came to those who were too visible. The inability to trust that keeps intimacy at arm's length once protected someone from the specific destruction that came from trusting the wrong person at the wrong time.

These patterns were intelligent. They were adaptive. They were the correct response to the specific threat environment of the person who first developed them.

They were handed to you without the original context. Without the original threat. Without any explanation of why this was supposed to be the way you moved through the world. Just the pattern itself, running in your nervous system like software installed before you knew you had a computer.

Looking at your most painful patterns through this lens does not make them acceptable to keep. It makes them comprehensible — and comprehensible is the prerequisite for changeable. You cannot update software you do not know you are running.

Reflection 8

You learned what love felt like from people who had not yet learned what love was.

The first template for love arrives before the first memory. In the quality of the earliest attachment — in whether the need was met or ignored or met inconsistently, in whether the environment was warm or cold or unpredictable, in whether the primary caregivers had the emotional capacity to see you as a separate person with separate needs or whether their own unprocessed pain required your emotional resources before you had fully developed your own.

Whatever that template was, it became the operating definition of love for your nervous system. Not the intellectual definition — not what you know love is supposed to be. The felt definition. The one your body uses to recognize love when it arrives. The one that determines which relationships feel real and which feel like something is missing.

If the template was love with conditions, you will feel most at home in conditional love. If the template was love that disappeared without warning, your nervous system will be most activated — most engaged, most present, most alive — in relationships where the possibility of disappearance is always present. If the template was love that required you to manage the other person's feelings to receive it, managing other people's feelings will feel like what intimacy looks like.

This is why the relationship that checked every intellectual box felt flat while the one that replicated the original wound felt electric. Electricity was what the original template produced. Your nervous system called it love because love was the first thing it felt that way about.

You are not condemned to repeat the template. But you are required to see it clearly — to understand that what you call chemistry and what the nervous system calls familiar are not always the same as what you actually need and deserve. The person who does not replicate the wound may initially feel boring. Stay long enough to find out if boring is actually safety. It frequently is.

Reflection 9

The child who survived by disappearing became the adult who disappears in every room she enters.

Disappearing is a skill. Do not underestimate what it took to develop it.

In environments where being seen was risky — where your needs made adults uncomfortable, where your presence required a performance that managed everyone else's emotional state, where the safest version of you was the quietest and most contained and least demanding version — becoming invisible was the most sophisticated coping mechanism available to a child with limited options.

You got very good at it. You learned to read the room before entering it. To assess what was needed from you and provide it before anyone had to ask. To shrink the parts of yourself that attracted unwanted attention and amplify the parts that produced warmth or approval or at least the absence of harm. You became an expert in other people's emotional landscapes and a stranger to your own.

And then you grew up and took the expertise with you.

The adult who disappears in rooms does not experience herself as hiding. She experiences herself as considerate. As easy to be around. As someone who does not make things complicated or require anything from anyone. These feel like virtues. They were virtues, in the original environment. They were the skills that got you through.

In adult life, they produce invisibility that masquerades as maturity. Needlessness that masquerades as self-sufficiency. The specific loneliness of a woman who is present everywhere and genuinely known nowhere, because the part of her that could be known has been so thoroughly managed into smallness that even she has lost reliable access to it.

The child who disappeared to survive deserved to be seen. Start seeing her now, even if no one else has yet learned to.

Reflection 10

Understanding where the wound came from does not erase it. But it stops you from blaming yourself for bleeding.

The origin story of your pain matters — not as an excuse that absolves you of responsibility for what you do with it, but as the specific antidote to the shame that has been compounding the original wound for most of your adult life.

Shame is the belief that the wound is evidence of something fundamentally wrong with you. That the patterns you carry are proof of a defect rather than an adaptation. That the way you respond to certain triggers, the relationships you have chosen, the places you have gotten stuck — that these things reveal something damning about your character rather than something comprehensible about your history.

The shame is often worse than the original wound. The wound happened to you. The shame you added afterward is the part you keep doing to yourself.

Understanding where it came from — really understanding, not as an intellectual exercise but as a felt recalibration of how you see your own story — removes the shame from the wound. What remains is the wound itself, which is significant and real and deserving of attention but is not, without the shame, unbearable.

People heal from extraordinary things when they are able to look at what happened to them with clarity rather than self-condemnation. The clarity is not comfortable. Seeing what actually happened, without the protective narrative of it was not that bad or I should be over this by now, requires a quality of honest self-witnessing that is among the more difficult things a person can do.

But on the other side of that honest witnessing is something the shame has been preventing: the specific self-compassion of someone who finally understands that they were doing the best they could with what they were given, in circumstances they did not choose, at an age when they had no other options.

You were not failing. You were surviving. Those two things deserve to be distinguished.

CHAPTER 3

What You Called Strength Was Often Just Endurance

The Difference Between Surviving and Actually Living

Reflection 11

Enduring what should have ended is not strength. It is loyalty to something that does not deserve it.

The cultural narrative around female strength is deeply confused on this point, and the confusion has cost women enormously. Staying has been rebranded as strength. Enduring has been rebranded as resilience. The woman who remains inside impossible circumstances without breaking has been celebrated as admirable when what she deserves is support in leaving.

Strength is not the absence of breaking points. Strength is not the capacity to absorb damage indefinitely without visible collapse. That is not strength. That is the specific suppression of a person who has learned that falling apart in front of other people is either unsafe or unfair to those around her, and who has therefore become extraordinary at metabolizing pain privately while presenting an intact surface to the world.

The woman who endures what should have ended is not strong in the way that actually serves her. She is loyal — to the relationship, the situation, the version of herself she has been inside that context, the hope that if she stays long enough something will finally shift. And loyalty is a beautiful quality in the right direction. Aimed at something that genuinely deserves it, loyalty produces profound and sustaining connection.

Aimed at your own suffering, it produces decades spent in what could have ended years earlier, if the cultural message about what strength looked like had been different. If someone had told you that leaving was not failure. That the strongest thing available to you was not absorbing more but refusing to.

You were not weak for staying. You were working with a definition of strength that did not include the option of your own protection. Update the definition. The strongest thing you can do right now may be the thing you have been convinced only weak women do.

Reflection 12

You wore your suffering like a badge because it was the only evidence you had that you were strong enough.

When external validation is unreliable — when the environment did not consistently reflect your worth back to you, when approval was conditional and withdrawn without warning, when you learned early that your value was contingent on performance rather than intrinsic to your existence — suffering becomes a strange kind of proof.

If I can handle this, I must be capable. If I am still standing after everything, I must be strong. If I have survived what would have broken other people, I must have something extraordinary in me.

All of that may be true. The problem is the logic that follows — the conclusion that because you can handle it, you should. That the capacity for endurance is an instruction to endure. That surviving something is evidence you were meant to stay inside it.

You were not meant to stay inside it. The capacity you developed for managing pain was a response to an environment that produced more pain than any person should be required to absorb. The capacity is real and it is impressive and it is yours. The thing that produced it was not necessary, not valuable, not the crucible that made you stronger in any way that justifies what it cost.

You do not need to keep earning the badge. You have already demonstrated, beyond any reasonable doubt, that you are capable of surviving extraordinary things. You are allowed to stop using your suffering as a test you keep passing. You have passed it. You can leave the examination room now.

Reflection 13

Resilience was supposed to be the bridge to something better. Not the destination you settled for.

Resilience has been so thoroughly celebrated in the conversation about mental health that something important has gotten lost: resilience is a means, not an end. The capacity to bounce back from adversity is valuable precisely because it enables movement — because it allows a person to recover from something difficult and continue toward something better.

When resilience becomes the end — when the goal becomes the ongoing capacity to absorb difficulty rather than the arrival at circumstances that no longer require it — something has gone quietly wrong. The bridge has been mistaken for the destination. The ability to survive the crossing has been confused with a reason to keep living on it.

This happens in relationships where the tolerance for pain is so high that the standard for acceptable keeps lowering. In work environments where the capacity for managing stress becomes license to keep piling it on. In internal life where the ability to carry more and more becomes the justification for never putting anything down.

Your resilience was developed for a purpose. That purpose was not to demonstrate indefinitely that you can absorb more. The purpose was to get you through something hard to somewhere better. If you are still in the hard thing — if the resilience has been running continuously for years without the somewhere better ever arriving — it is not because you are not resilient enough.

It is because resilience alone cannot move you. Only choice moves you. And the choice to stop treating the bridge as home is available to you right now.

Reflection 14

Some versions of toughness are just numbness with better posture.

The distinction is felt, not observed. From the outside, the woman who has genuinely processed her difficulty and the woman who has simply gone numb to it can look identical. Both are functional. Both are composed. Both continue moving through their lives without visible evidence of the weight they carry.

From the inside, the difference is everything.

Genuine resilience has feeling in it. The woman who has done the actual work of processing what happened to her has access to the full range of her emotional life — including joy that is not contaminated by waiting for it to be taken away, intimacy that is not held at a managed distance, the ordinary pleasures of an ordinary day that land fully rather than sliding past a surface that has learned not to let things in.

Numbness looks like peace from the outside. Inside, it is the specific flatness of someone who learned that feeling cost too much and stopped allowing the full frequency. The aliveness got turned down along with the pain. The capacity for genuine pleasure narrowed alongside the capacity for genuine grief. The armor that was installed to manage the wound ended up managing everything — not just the painful things but the beautiful ones too.

Ask yourself honestly: are you genuinely okay, or have you simply become very good at not feeling how not okay you are? The question is not comfortable. The answer is necessary. Because you cannot heal what you have learned not to feel. And you deserve to feel everything — not just the pain, which has been available in abundance, but the full, unmanaged, unarmored range of being a person who is actually alive inside her own life.

Reflection 15

The strongest thing you will ever do is admit something is not working and stop pretending it is.

The pretending takes extraordinary energy. The maintenance of fine — the continuous construction and presentation of a surface that reads as functional, as capable, as someone who has her life together — is one of the most exhausting things a human being can do, and it is so normalized among women who grew up learning to manage their environments that the exhaustion has become background noise. Just the cost of existing. Just what it takes to get through the day.

But examine what the energy of that pretending could produce if it were freed. The cognitive load of managing two simultaneous realities — the one that is true and the one that is presented — is immense. The emotional labor of performing okayness while something else is actually happening occupies resources that belong to everything else. The creative energy, the relational presence, the capacity for genuine engagement with the actual texture of your days — all of it is being taxed by the performance.

Admitting that something is not working does not make it worse. The thing was already not working. The admission simply stops adding the cost of the pretending to the existing cost of the problem. It is the specific relief of setting down something heavy you had convinced yourself you were not carrying.

It will feel vulnerable. It may feel like failure — like the acknowledgment that you have not, in fact, been handling it as well as you have been presenting. Let it feel that way. The feeling is temporary. The freedom available on the other side of the honest admission is not.

The strongest women in any room are rarely the ones who look most composed. They are the ones who have been honest enough with themselves about what is not working to stop pouring their energy into maintaining the appearance that it is.

That honesty is available to you right now. It was always the most powerful move on the board.

CHAPTER 4

The Stories You Told to Keep the Suffering in Place

The Narratives That Justified Staying in What Was Hurting You

Reflection 16

Every story you told yourself about why you had to stay was a story that kept you from leaving.

The stories are sophisticated. They have to be — they are constructed by a highly intelligent person who needed them to be airtight enough to hold up against the persistent inner voice that kept raising its hand and pointing at the door.

He will change. The timing is not right. I have invested too much to leave now. It will affect the children. I do not know who I am without this. It is not that bad. Other people have it worse. Maybe I am the problem. Maybe if I were different, this would work. Maybe I just need to try harder, communicate better, understand more, give it more time.

Each story is built from some genuine material. Real complexity, real love, real legitimate concern for the people involved. The stories are not lies, exactly. They are selections — the specific details that support remaining, assembled into a coherent narrative and reinforced every time the instinct toward leaving gets loud enough to require management.

What is left out of the story is equally selected. The cost that keeps accumulating. The version of yourself that has been getting smaller inside this situation for years. The answer to the honest question of what you would tell a woman you loved who described your exact circumstances to you.

You already know what you would tell her.

The story you told yourself was not the truth. It was the construction of someone who needed a reason to stay in a place that felt more survivable than the unknown outside it. The construction was understandable. The cost of maintaining it has been your actual life.

What would happen if you stopped needing the story?

Reflection 17

You convinced yourself you were fine because the alternative — admitting you were not — required action you were not ready to take.

Fine is the most consequential lie in the English language when it is directed inward. Not because the word itself is damaging. Because of what maintaining it requires — the ongoing suppression of the accurate internal report in favor of the manageable one. The daily decision to file not fine under irrelevant rather than under urgent.

The specific genius of convincing yourself you are fine is that it removes the pressure of having to do something about not being fine. If you are fine, no action is required. If you are fine, the situation does not need to change. If you are fine, the investment you have made in the current arrangement is not in jeopardy and the terrifying uncertainty of a different life does not have to be confronted.

The problem is that not fine does not respond to being filed as fine. It simply goes somewhere else — into the body, into the specific inflammation of chronic stress, into the exhaustion that sleep does not fix and the resentment that arrives without clear cause and the background anxiety of someone whose internal alarm system has been ignored so many times it has started producing a continuous low-level signal rather than acute alarms that might require a response.

The admission that you are not fine is not the catastrophe the fine-maintenance has been protecting you from. It is the beginning of being actually fine — eventually, through the work that the honest admission makes possible. The catastrophe is not the admission. The catastrophe is another decade of fine that costs you everything while producing nothing.

You are allowed to not be fine. It is, in fact, the most honest thing available to you right now.

Reflection 18

The story that you deserved what you received was not the truth. It was the conclusion of someone in too much pain to see clearly.

Children who are harmed by their caregivers almost universally conclude that they deserved the harm. Not because this conclusion is logical — it is not — but because the alternative is more terrifying. If the person who was supposed to protect me chose to harm me, the world is not safe and I have no reliable source of protection. But if I somehow caused or deserved the harm, then the world has rules and I can learn to follow them and stay safe.

The child's conclusion was a survival mechanism. The adult's continuation of that conclusion is the original wound's most lasting damage.

You did not deserve what happened to you. Not the childhood that asked too much of you. Not the relationship that diminished you. Not the dynamic that required your smallness as the condition of belonging. Not the treatment you received from people who were working out their own unprocessed pain on the most available and most forgiving person in the room.

The story that you deserved it has been functioning as a cage with the door left open. It keeps you in relationships that replicate the original harm because if you deserved it then, you deserve it now. It keeps you from demanding better because demanding better requires the belief that better is something you are entitled to. It keeps the suffering in place because the suffering feels, at some level below conscious thought, like the appropriate consequence of being the kind of person who deserves suffering.

You are not that kind of person. There is no kind of person who deserves suffering. The story was wrong from the beginning. And you are allowed to stop living inside a narrative that was built by a child in pain to make an unsafe world feel navigable.

Reflection 19

Hope is not a reason to stay in something harmful. Hope that requires your destruction to survive is not hope. It is delay.

Hope has been weaponized against women in painful situations with extraordinary efficiency. Not by malicious design, necessarily — but by the specific cultural reverence for staying, for trying harder, for being the person who does not give up, for believing in people and relationships and the possibility of change even when the evidence has been consistently pointing in a different direction for years.

The hope is real. The love underneath it is often real. The desire for the thing to be different is genuine and human and entirely understandable. Nobody wants to grieve a relationship or a life they built inside an investment of years and care and genuine longing for something good.

But hope requires a reasonable basis. Hope based on actual evidence of change — on behavioral shifts that have held across time, not promises made in the aftermath of damage — is legitimate and deserves its place in the decision. Hope based on the sheer force of wanting something to be different, in the absence of any evidence that it is moving in that direction, is not hope. It is the specific cruelty of keeping yourself tethered to something that has already shown you what it is.

Something can show you what it is and you can still love it. Love and clear seeing are not mutually exclusive. But love that requires you to stop seeing clearly is not love protecting you. It is the fear of grief wearing love's clothing.

You are allowed to grieve what something was not while clearly seeing what it was. That grief is not defeat. It is the most honest act of love available — for yourself, and ultimately for everyone involved.

Reflection 20

The story ends when you stop needing it to justify the suffering.

Every narrative has a function. The story you have been telling about your suffering — why it was necessary, why it made you stronger, why it was not as bad as it seems, why you could not have done differently, why the people involved deserve more understanding than the harm they caused would suggest — that story has been performing a specific and important service.

It has been making the unbearable bearable. It has been providing structure around experiences that, without the narrative scaffolding, would feel too chaotic, too random, too cruel in their arbitrariness to be survived. The story gave the suffering meaning. And meaning, even constructed meaning, is one of the most powerful pain-management tools available to a human mind.

Viktor Frankl observed from inside a Nazi concentration camp that the people most likely to survive were not the physically strongest. They were the ones who could construct meaning from the experience — who could locate some purpose or future or reason inside the suffering that made the suffering survivable.

The story was your version of that construction. It served you. Honor it for what it gave you.

And then ask whether you still need it. Because the story that made the suffering survivable is also the story that keeps the suffering in place — that makes it meaningful enough to maintain, purposeful enough to justify, understandable enough not to leave. And you are not in the concentration camp anymore. The circumstances that made the story necessary have changed or can change or you can change in relation to them.

The story ends when you no longer need suffering to have a reason to exist. When your life is no longer organized around the meaning you extracted from your pain. When the wound has been honestly acknowledged and grieved and integrated — not resolved neatly, but no longer requiring a narrative to make it tolerable.

That ending is not a loss. It is the space where your actual life, the one that was always waiting on the other side of the story you needed to stop telling, finally gets room to begin.

***

"She had been the author of a story that kept her inside a life she had outgrown. The day she put down the pen was the day the real story could finally start."

PART TWO: THE WAYS YOU BETRAY YOURSELF

The Daily, Quiet, Accumulated Acts of Self-Abandonment

CHAPTER 5

The Betrayal That Happens in Small Moments

How Self-Abandonment Operates Below the Level of Drama

Reflection 21

Self-betrayal rarely arrives as a single catastrophic decision. It accumulates in moments so small you barely notice them.

Nobody wakes up and decides to abandon themselves. The decision does not come with a timestamp or a clear memory of the moment it happened. What happens instead is a thousand micro-moments across years — each one so small it barely registers as a choice, each one so reasonable in isolation that the pattern they form together stays invisible until the accumulated weight of it becomes impossible to carry without noticing.

The moment you stayed quiet when something needed to be said. The moment you rearranged your schedule around someone who would not have rearranged theirs around you. The moment your instinct said something is wrong here and you talked yourself out of it within thirty seconds because acting on it felt harder than ignoring it. The moment you apologized for taking up space in a room you had every right to be in.

None of these moments felt like betrayal. They felt like consideration, or practicality, or the reasonable management of a life with competing demands. They felt like maturity. Like not being difficult. Like being the kind of person who does not make everything about herself.

But add them up. Really add them up — across a week, a month, a decade of small moments where the version of yourself that needed something consistently got moved to the back of the line. What you get is not consideration. What you get is a woman who has systematically deprioritized her own experience until she is genuinely uncertain whether her experience counts.

The accumulation is the damage. And the damage becomes visible not in a single dramatic moment but in the exhaustion that has no specific cause, the resentment that arrives without a clear target, the hollow feeling of a life that is full of activity and empty of genuine self.

The self-betrayal was not a single event you can point to and address. It is a pattern that has to be interrupted at the level of the small moments — in the next one, and the one after that, and the one after that.

Reflection 22

Every time you dismissed your own instinct to defer to someone else's certainty, you made a withdrawal from your self-trust account.

The account is probably significantly overdrawn by now.

Your instincts were not wrong. They were inconvenient — for other people, for the arrangement that depended on your compliance, for the version of events that required your doubt in order to hold together. The gaslighting did not always come from other people. A great deal of it was self-administered, practiced so consistently in the service of managing relationships that the habit of overriding your own knowing became indistinguishable from humility.

Humility says: I might be wrong, let me consider other perspectives. Self-betrayal says: I am definitely wrong, and whoever is most certain in this room is the one I should believe instead of myself.

Think about the times you knew. The relationship that had a specific feeling in your body from the first month that you explained away for three years. The friend whose energy shifted around your good news in a way you registered and immediately found a generous interpretation for. The work environment whose culture revealed itself in the first week and that you convinced yourself you were misreading. The body that was sending signals you categorized as anxiety rather than accuracy.

You knew. You knew considerably more than you acted on, and considerably earlier than you were willing to admit. And every time you overrode the knowing — every time you chose someone else's version of events over your own direct perception — you added another entry to the ledger of evidence that your perception cannot be trusted.

The account can be rebuilt. It is rebuilt the same way it was depleted — one small moment at a time. The next time you know something, let yourself know it. You do not have to act on it immediately. Just stop arguing with yourself about whether you are allowed to perceive what you are perceiving.

Reflection 23

The apology you did not owe. The boundary you set and immediately took back. The need you swallowed because the timing felt wrong. That is where the betrayal lives.

Not in the enormous failures. In these.

The apology that arrived before anyone asked for it, issued preemptively to manage the emotional atmosphere of a room where you had done nothing wrong except exist in a way that might inconvenience someone. The sorry that came out of your mouth reflexively, trained by years of environments where your presence required apology as the price of admission.

The boundary that held for four days before the other person's discomfort became your emergency. The limit you set from a genuine place that you began walking back the moment the resistance arrived — softening it, qualifying it, finding the version that caused the least friction until what remained was so diluted it no longer functioned as a limit at all.

The need — for rest, for acknowledgment, for time, for the basic reciprocity of a relationship that moves in both directions — that you swallowed because right now was never the right time, because someone else needed something more urgent, because your need seemed smaller than the cost of expressing it and so it went back down and settled somewhere in your body to wait.

Each of these is a small act of self-erasure. Each one, in isolation, seems reasonable and even generous. Together, over years, they constitute a systematic practice of treating yourself as the least important person in every room you enter.

The correction is not dramatic. It is the next apology you do not give for something that does not deserve one. The next boundary you hold through the discomfort of someone else's resistance. The next need you name out loud before it gets swallowed.

Reflection 24

You became an expert at talking yourself out of what you clearly knew because knowing it required doing something about it.

The not-knowing was a choice. Possibly the most consequential choice being made in your life, and possibly the one most dressed up as something else — as open-mindedness, as giving people the benefit of the doubt, as refusing to be the kind of woman who jumps to conclusions or makes things difficult when they could be smooth.

But underneath the benefit of the doubt was something more specific and more honest. Knowing what you knew would have required you to act on it. And acting on it would have required changes — to the relationship, to the arrangement, to the story you had been telling about your life and the people in it. Changes that were frightening. Changes that would cost you the familiar, whatever the familiar was costing you in return.

So you developed remarkable skill at the internal argument. At taking the clear perception and immediately submitting it to a tribunal of alternative explanations. Maybe I am reading too much into it. Maybe I am projecting. Maybe I am too sensitive. Maybe this is my anxiety, not information. Maybe I should wait and see. Maybe I am not being fair.

The maybe is where the knowing goes to die. The maybe is the space between perception and action where enough doubt can be manufactured to make inaction feel like wisdom rather than avoidance.

You were not uncertain. You were afraid of what certainty required. The distinction matters because uncertainty is addressed by gathering more information, and what you needed was not more information. What you needed was the courage to act on what you already had.

The certainty is still there. It has been waiting under every maybe you have stacked on top of it.

Reflection 25

The most dangerous betrayals are not the dramatic ones. They are the quiet daily ones that never even feel like choices.

Dramatic betrayals are at least visible. They produce a crisis that demands a response. They make the damage undeniable and the need for change impossible to defer.

Quiet betrayals produce nothing so useful. They produce gradual erosion — the slow, daily, undetected wearing away of the self that happens when the pattern is too normalized to trigger alarm. The woman who has been quietly betraying herself for years does not look like someone in crisis. She looks functional. She looks busy. She looks like she is handling everything, which she is, which is precisely the problem.

The crisis that forces change requires the damage to become acute. The quiet betrayal keeps the damage chronic — present and accumulating but never quite severe enough to override the enormous effort of changing, never quite unbearable enough to make the unfamiliarity of a different life feel worth the cost of getting there.

The quiet betrayals are the ones worth paying attention to. Not because they each individually constitute catastrophe, but because they constitute the actual texture of your relationship with yourself — the daily evidence, accumulated over years, of whether you are someone who matters to yourself.

Start noticing them. Not to judge them. To count them. Because the count, when you actually run it, tends to be the thing that makes the change feel necessary rather than optional.

CHAPTER 6

Staying When You Knew You Should Leave

The Specific Cost of Remaining in What No Longer Serves You

Reflection 26

You did not stay because you did not know. You stayed because leaving required a version of yourself you had not yet built.

The knowledge was there. Earlier than you wanted it to be, probably. That quiet, persistent awareness in the background of everything that this was not right, this was not what you needed, this was not somewhere you could stay indefinitely and survive with yourself intact. The awareness arrived and you noted it and you filed it under not yet and kept going.

Not yet is honest. Not yet acknowledges the knowing while also acknowledging what the knowing would cost — and what it would require. Leaving requires a self who believes she can survive the aftermath. Who trusts that the unknown on the other side of leaving, however uncertain, is survivable. Who has enough internal resource to tolerate the grief of ending something, the anxiety of starting something new, the specific disorientation of building a life that does not have the familiar painful thing at its center.

If you did not have that self yet, staying was not stupidity. It was the reasonable behavior of someone who was not yet equipped for the alternative. The problem is when not yet becomes permanent — when the building of the self who can leave keeps getting deferred because the not yet has become its own kind of home.

You build that self not by waiting until you feel ready — ready almost never arrives before the move — but by taking the first small step from inside the feeling of not being ready. By doing the thing before the resource feels sufficient and discovering, through the doing, that you were more capable than the staying had allowed you to believe.

The version of you who could have left sooner was built inside the leaving. She was always going to be built there. The only question was when you would begin.

Reflection 27

Every day you stayed past the moment you knew was one more day of evidence — to yourself — that you did not believe you could survive without it.

This is the hidden cost that never makes it into the accounting. Not just what the situation cost you in terms of time and energy and opportunity and the specific version of yourself that was available there. But what remaining in it, past the moment you knew, taught you about your own assessment of your worth and your capability.

Every day of staying was a vote. A vote, cast in behavior rather than words, for the proposition that whatever was on the other side of leaving was more frightening than what you were currently inside. That the familiar painful thing was preferable to the unknown better thing. That you could not be trusted to survive a life that did not include this arrangement, this relationship, this version of yourself organized around managing what was wrong.

The votes accumulate into a verdict. Not delivered externally — you deliver it to yourself, below conscious awareness, through the pattern of your choices. And the verdict becomes the operating belief: I cannot survive without this. I am not the kind of person who can do the thing that leaving requires. I have too much invested to start again. I am not strong enough, brave enough, worth enough to choose better.

None of these verdicts are accurate. All of them feel true because they have been built from real evidence — the evidence of your own repeated behavior — rather than from someone else's assessment.

You can begin overturning the verdict today. Not with a declaration, not with a decision made in an emotional moment that does not survive contact with ordinary Tuesday. With the next vote cast differently. And then the next. Until the evidence starts pointing somewhere else.

Reflection 28

The sunk cost of what you have already given is not a reason to keep giving. It is a reason to grieve what it cost you and go.

Behavioral economists have a name for what keeps people inside situations they should leave long after the evidence has made leaving clearly preferable. The sunk cost fallacy — the irrational but deeply human tendency to continue investing in something not because of its future value but because of the past investment already made. The logic says: I have given so much that leaving now would mean all of that was wasted.

The logic is wrong. Not morally wrong — emotionally it makes complete sense, and most people who reason this way are not being irrational in the colloquial sense but are responding to a very real psychological pain. The sunk cost logic is wrong because the past investment does not change the future return. The years already spent in something that was not working do not transform that something into something that will work if you simply continue. The cost already paid does not become worthwhile by paying more.

What it does become is a grief. The years, the energy, the love, the hope, the version of yourself you were while inside this — those are a real loss. They deserve genuine mourning. The grief is not a stage to rush through on the way to moving on. It is the necessary acknowledgment that something real was spent on something that did not return the investment.

Grieve it fully. Give the loss its proper weight without using the weight of it to justify remaining inside what caused it. The grief and the leaving are not in conflict. They happen together — the mourning of what was given and the decision that no more will be given without better return.

Reflection 29

Leaving does not mean the love was not real. It means you finally loved yourself as much as you loved what was hurting you.

The cultural narrative around staying conflates love with endurance in ways that damage people who are genuinely loving and genuinely suffering simultaneously. The belief that if the love is real, you stay. That leaving is evidence the love was insufficient. That the willingness to remain inside something damaging is the measure of the love's authenticity.

This belief keeps people inside things that are hurting them out of a genuine desire to prove the realness of their love. And the love often is real. Loving someone who is not good for you is one of the most human experiences available. The two things — genuine love and genuine incompatibility, genuine love and genuine harm — are not mutually exclusive. They coexist constantly, in ordinary people's lives, producing the specific suffering of someone who cannot simply fall out of love with what is hurting her because the love is not a decision that responds to logical instruction.

What changes is not the love. What changes is the priority. Leaving is not the withdrawal of love for the other person. It is the extension of love to yourself — the decision that you are also someone whose experience matters, whose wellbeing is also a priority, who also deserves protection from harm even when the harm comes from something you love.

You can love someone and leave them. You can grieve the loss genuinely, without the grief meaning the leaving was wrong. You can hold the love and the departure simultaneously without needing one to cancel the other.

The love was real. It was not enough reason to stay. Both of those things are true at the same time.

Reflection 30

Whatever you are holding onto that you have outgrown — the relationship, the identity, the version of yourself built inside the wound — it is standing between you and something that actually fits.

Outgrowing something is not a judgment of its worth. The shoe that fit perfectly at twenty was not a bad shoe. It simply stopped fitting when the foot grew. Continuing to wear it after that point is not loyalty to the shoe or evidence of love for the journey you walked together. It is the specific daily damage of forcing yourself into something designed for a smaller version of who you are.

You have grown. Whether through the deliberate work of self-examination or simply through the accumulation of lived experience, the version of you that exists right now is not identical to the version that entered the thing you are holding onto. Your needs have evolved. Your understanding of what you deserve has deepened — or is in the process of deepening. Your capacity for honest self-assessment has expanded. The thing that fit when you entered it may not fit the person you have become inside it.

Holding onto it is not preventing the growth. The growth has already happened. What it is preventing is the ability to move into the life that corresponds to who you have grown into. The life that fits this version — not the smaller, earlier, less self-aware version, but the current one.

That life is not a fantasy. It exists on the other side of the releasing. Not perfectly assembled and waiting for your arrival, but possible — genuinely, specifically possible — in ways that the current arrangement makes structurally unavailable.

Let go of the shoe that stopped fitting. Not because it was a bad shoe. Because your feet are bigger now.

CHAPTER 7

The Lies You Told Yourself to Make the Pain Bearable

Internal Deception as a Coping Mechanism and Its Hidden Cost

Reflection 31

The lie was never meant to be permanent. It was a bridge. You just never got off it.

Protective narratives are not character failures. They are psychological infrastructure — built in moments when the truth was more than what the available resources could support, when honest reckoning with what was happening would have required either action or collapse, and neither was accessible. The lie that made things bearable was the bridge that got you across something you were not equipped to cross fully aware.

The problem is not that the bridge was built. The problem is that bridges are not homes. They are temporary structures designed to get you from one bank to another — not to be inhabited indefinitely while both banks wait.

At some point the bridge became the location. The temporary reckoning-postponement became the permanent operating reality. The narrative — he is trying, she means well, it is getting better, I am fine, this is just how things are — stopped being the thing that got you through the hard stretch and became the wallpaper of your life. Present so constantly that you stopped registering it as a constructed story and started accepting it as simply the truth.

The way off the bridge is not to condemn the lie. The lie was intelligent. The way off is to ask what truth the bridge was built to avoid and whether you are now capable of standing on that truth without the bridge's support. You are almost certainly more capable of it than you were when the bridge was first constructed. The crossing will still be uncomfortable. Bridges exist because crossings are uncomfortable.

But you were not meant to live on it. The other bank is where you were always going.

Reflection 32

He will change. She means well. It will get better. Things will calm down. You said these things enough times that they stopped being hopes and became the plan.

Hope is healthy. Hope directed at genuine evidence of movement is one of the most sustaining psychological resources available to a person navigating difficult circumstances. The hope that keeps you going through a genuine rough patch in a relationship that is fundamentally sound is not the same thing as the hope that keeps you tethered to a situation that has been consistently telling you something different for years.

The distinction is not about the feeling. The feeling of hope is identical in both cases — warm, sustaining, oriented toward a better future that feels genuinely possible. The distinction is about the evidence. One hope is supported by actual change — behavioral, sustained, independent of whether you are watching. The other is supported by the desire for change and the fear of what losing hope would require.

When the hope becomes the plan — when I hope this will improve becomes I am staying because this will improve, without any particular evidence that improvement is in progress — the hope has shifted from a sustaining resource to a structural dependency. The situation depends on your continued hope to remain tolerable. And your hope depends on not looking too clearly at the evidence that has been accumulating.

Allowing yourself to look clearly does not kill the hope if the hope has genuine basis. It only kills the hope that was manufactured in the absence of basis. And hope manufactured without basis is not hope. It is the specific cruelty of a story that keeps you where you are while the time it costs keeps passing.

Reflection 33

Optimism about unchanging situations is not hope. It is the specific cruelty of keeping yourself attached to something that has shown you clearly who it is.

Maya Angelou said it with a precision that has never been improved upon: when someone shows you who they are, believe them the first time.

You were probably shown much earlier than the first time you were willing to believe. Not because you are naive — you are not naive. Because believing what you were shown required a response that the belief was not yet supported by enough internal resource to produce.

The situation showed you what it was. The person showed you what they were capable of and what they were not. The dynamic revealed its structure through the pattern of how it consistently operated rather than through the exceptions that punctuated the pattern. And you saw it. You registered it. You felt the accuracy of the perception in your body before your mind found the explanation that made staying feel reasonable.

And then you optimized. You focused on the exceptions. You found the most generous interpretation of the data. You built a case, constructed from real pieces but assembled selectively, for why the pattern was not what it appeared to be and why the next iteration would be different.

This is not stupidity. It is the specific intelligence of a person who needed the situation to be different from what it was and applied her considerable cognitive resources to building the case for it. The intelligence is not the problem. The application of it to the project of not-seeing is.

Believe what you have been shown. Not cynically — with the honest reckoning of someone who is finally allowing the full picture to be as large as it actually is.

Reflection 34

You are allowed to see someone you love clearly without the clarity destroying the love. But the clarity must be allowed to exist.

The fear underneath most willful not-seeing in relationships is this: if I see this person clearly — if I allow myself to acknowledge what they are consistently doing, what they are not capable of, what the pattern has been showing me — the love will not survive the clarity. And losing the love is more frightening than maintaining the distortion.

So the distortion is maintained. The full picture is kept partial. The evidence is managed into a shape that allows love to continue without having to reckon with what loving this person in this way is actually costing you.

But love and clear vision are not mutually exclusive. They can coexist — and in genuinely healthy relationships, they do coexist. Loving someone clearly means seeing their actual character rather than the curated version the story requires. It means allowing the disappointments and limitations to be real alongside the genuine warmth and genuine history. It means being in relationship with an actual person rather than the version of them that the hope has constructed.

Sometimes the clear vision confirms that the love is enough and the relationship is worth continuing. Sometimes the clear vision reveals that the love, while genuine, is not sufficient to make the relationship sustainable — that loving someone does not obligate you to organize your life around what they cannot give you.

The clarity does not destroy the love. It simply places the love in an accurate context. What you do with the love inside that accurate context is a separate and subsequent question. But it cannot be answered honestly from inside the distortion.

Let yourself see.

Reflection 35

The moment you stopped needing the lie, you did not lose anything. You just stopped paying the cost of maintaining it.

The maintenance of a protective narrative requires enormous ongoing energy. The constant editing of incoming information to fit the approved version of events. The management of your own perceptions — the daily internal negotiation between what you are directly experiencing and what the story requires you to experience instead. The specific vigilance of someone who cannot afford to let the evidence become too visible lest it overwhelm the narrative that is making everything manageable.

When the narrative finally drops — when you stop needing it because you have developed enough internal resource to stand on the truth without it — what releases is not the love, not the history, not the genuine parts of the experience that deserved to be what you needed them to be.

What releases is the effort. The cognitive load of the management. The specific exhaustion of a mind that has been doing two jobs simultaneously — experiencing reality and immediately translating it into the acceptable version.

People describe this drop as loss, initially, because the story was a structure and structures feel like something when they are removed even if what they were doing was constraining rather than supporting. What follows the feeling of loss, when it is allowed to settle, is something much closer to relief. The specific lightness of someone who has put down something heavy and discovered that their shoulders were designed for a different load.

You do not lose anything when the lie ends except the cost of telling it. And the cost was your own clarity, your own energy, your own relationship with your direct perception of your life.

Those are not things you could afford to keep losing.

CHAPTER 8

What You Accepted Because You Did Not Know You Could Ask for More

The Role of Low Expectations in Sustained Self-Betrayal

Reflection 36

You accepted less because you had been given less for so long that less started to feel like enough.

Standards do not exist in isolation. They are calibrated against experience — against what has been consistently available, what has been reliably received, what has been present often enough to constitute the baseline from which more and less are measured.

When the baseline is set low enough, for long enough, the baseline becomes the ceiling. What would have been clearly insufficient to someone with a different reference point becomes the definition of enough for the person whose entire experience of relationships, love, or care has been lived within a narrow and insufficient range.

This is not stupidity. It is the perfectly logical result of calibration against available data. The woman who grew up with conditional love does not choose conditional love as an adult because she lacks self-respect. She gravitates toward it because it matches the template she has for what love feels like. The woman who was given inconsistent attention does not choose unreliable partners because something is wrong with her. She chooses them because reliability does not feel as recognizable as inconsistency.

The recalibration is the work. Not simply being told you deserve more — that information, while true, does not automatically upgrade the felt sense of what enough looks like. The recalibration happens through the sustained experience of actually receiving more. Of staying in the discomfort of being loved consistently until consistent love registers as real rather than suspect. Of noticing when the old template pulls and choosing against it deliberately, repeatedly, until a new template begins to form.

You deserve more. Knowing that is the beginning. Learning what more actually feels like inside your body is the work.

Reflection 37

Your baseline for what love looks like was set by the first people who loved you. If they loved you poorly, you learned to accept poor love.

John Bowlby spent decades documenting what is now one of the most robust findings in developmental psychology: the patterns of early attachment become the templates through which all subsequent attachment is experienced. Not just influenced. Templated. The way the earliest caregiving felt — its consistency, its warmth, its reliability, its capacity to receive the child's full emotional range — becomes the operating definition of what love feels like at the level of the nervous system, below conscious preference and intellectual understanding.

This means that if the early love was inconsistent, inconsistency feels like love. If the early love required your performance, love requiring your performance feels familiar. If the early love was present in the good moments and withdrew in the difficult ones, you will be most drawn to the specific emotional signature of warmth-contingent-on-behavior because that is the signature your nervous system filed under what love is.

You did not choose this template. It was installed before you could read, before you could evaluate what was being given to you, before you had any reference point that would have allowed you to recognize it as insufficient.

But you are reading now. You have reference points now — in what you know about healthy relationships, in what you have glimpsed in other people's connections, in the occasional experience of being genuinely cared for that produced a feeling unfamiliar enough to register as different.

The template can be updated. Not quickly and not without the specific disorientation of a nervous system encountering something different from what it expects. But updated — through experience, through therapy, through the deliberate choice to stay long enough in what is actually good to let it become familiar.

Reflection 38

Gratitude for crumbs is not a virtue when you deserved the whole thing.

Gratitude is one of the most consistently beneficial psychological practices available — when it is directed at genuine abundance. When it is directed at insufficiency, gratitude becomes a tool of self-management rather than genuine appreciation. It becomes the mechanism by which you talk yourself into being satisfied with what is not enough so that you do not have to face the discomfort of wanting what is not being given.

You were probably taught to be grateful. To see the good. To focus on what is there rather than what is missing. These are genuinely valuable orientations when they are applied to life's genuine goods. When they are applied to relationships that are consistently giving you less than you need, they become the specific mechanism of your own accommodation — the way you manage your own expectations into submission so the gap between what you need and what you are receiving does not become intolerable enough to require action.

Gratitude for what is genuinely there is appropriate. Gratitude manufactured to suppress the legitimate recognition that what is there is not enough is not gratitude. It is the spiritual bypassing of your own accurate assessment.

You are allowed to acknowledge what is good and simultaneously acknowledge that what is good is not sufficient. You are allowed to appreciate the crumbs and still name clearly that you deserved the whole thing. The naming is not ingratitude. It is the honest recognition that your hunger was real and legitimate and was not adequately fed — and that recognizing this is not a character failure but the beginning of being willing to seek what will actually fill you.

Reflection 39

The moment you raise your standard is the moment you discover which relationships were built to meet it and which were counting on you never to.

Raising your standard is not a declaration of war. It is not a demand for perfection or an ultimatum issued in an emotional moment. It is the quiet, internal shift of the line — the recalibration of what you are willing to accept and what you are not, communicated not necessarily through announcement but through the pattern of your behavior. Through what you continue to accept and what you no longer do. Through what you name instead of swallowing. Through the specific evidence of a woman who has updated her understanding of what she deserves and is beginning to live from that update.

What the shift reveals is immediate and usually surprising in its clarity. The relationships that had genuine substance beneath them — that were not entirely constructed on your willingness to accept less — respond to your raised standard with adjustment. Perhaps not perfectly, perhaps not without friction and negotiation and the discomfort of both people recalibrating. But with the fundamental willingness of someone who wants to be in relationship with you at the level you are now operating from.

The relationships that were constructed entirely on your low expectations respond differently. They push back. They call the standard unreasonable. They reference who you used to be with a nostalgia that is actually a complaint. They find ways to communicate that your growth is the problem — that the version of you who expected less was more loveable than the version who expects what she deserves.

That communication is the clearest possible signal. The relationship that requires your smallness to function was never going to give you what you needed. You were never going to get there by staying inside it and hoping it would become something it was not designed to be.

Raise the standard. Let the clarity come. It is the most useful information available.

Reflection 40

You are not too much for the life you actually want. You were just surrounded by people who benefited from convincing you that you were.

Too much is one of the most damaging phrases in the emotional vocabulary of women who have grown up in environments that needed their reduction. Not because the phrase was always stated directly — though sometimes it was. But because the message was delivered through the specific quality of the response to your full self. Through the withdrawal of warmth when you were too loud, too emotional, too ambitious, too certain, too present in a room that found your presence inconvenient.

You learned to read the too much signal the way you learned to read every other signal in an environment that required your hypervigilance. You learned where the line was. And you began, with the quiet efficiency of someone who has understood that adjustment is required for survival, to stay reliably on the acceptable side of it.

The problem is that the line was not objective. The line was drawn by people who benefited from your smallness. Who were more comfortable with a reduced version of you because the full version required something from them — more space, more reciprocity, more genuine presence — that they were either unwilling or unable to provide. The line was a preference masquerading as a fact. A self-serving assessment presented as the truth about who you are.

The life you want does not have that line. The people in it do not require your reduction as the condition of your belonging. The relationships, the work, the daily experience of being yourself without calculating what percentage of yourself is currently safe to express — those exist. Not as fantasy. As the actual lives of women who stopped accepting the too much verdict and discovered, gradually and then suddenly, that the right people find the full version of them not too much but exactly enough.

You were never too much. You were with people who were too small to hold you.

That is a very different problem. And unlike being too much — which, if true, would be yours to fix — it is not yours to solve.

***

"She spent years making herself smaller for people who were never going to grow large enough to deserve her. The day she stopped shrinking was the day she finally found out what she was actually made of."

PART THREE: THE TRUTH ABOUT YOUR PAIN

What Your Suffering Has Been Trying to Tell You

CHAPTER 9

Your Pain Has Been Speaking. You Stopped Listening.

What the Suffering Was Actually Communicating

Reflection 41

Pain is the most honest thing you have. It does not lie. It does not perform. It simply arrives at what is wrong before your conscious mind gets there.

Every other signal in your life can be managed. Your face can perform fine when nothing is fine. Your words can deliver the acceptable version of events when the actual version is considerably more complicated. Your behavior can maintain the appearance of a person who is handling everything when what is actually happening is that everything is handling her.

Pain cannot be managed that way. It arrives before the performance has time to assemble. It shows up in the body before the mind has agreed to acknowledge it — in the stomach that contracts when a certain person calls, in the chest that tightens around a conversation before a single word has been exchanged, in the specific heaviness that descends on Sunday evenings before a week you have not consciously admitted you are dreading.

The body does not have access to your protective narratives. It does not receive the edited version. It receives the direct signal — the unmediated, unspun, accurate assessment of the situation — and it responds accordingly, with the specific physiological signatures of threat and safety and loss and grief that the performance upstairs has been carefully not acknowledging.

This is not a design flaw. This is your most reliable compass, running underneath the stories you tell yourself and the stories you tell everyone else, pointing at what is actually true when everything else is pointing at what is convenient.

The pain was not random. It was not a malfunction. It was not anxiety that needed to be managed or sensitivity that needed to be toughened or irrationality that needed to be reasoned through. It was information, arriving in the most direct form available, about something real that needed your attention.

How long has it been speaking? How long have you been responding by turning down the volume?

Reflection 42

The anxiety is not the enemy. It is the alarm. The problem is what the alarm has been going off about — and the fact that you turned it down instead of addressing the fire.

Anxiety has a terrible reputation. In a culture that values composure and productivity and the specific kind of functional calm that allows people to continue moving through systems that are not working, anxiety gets framed as the problem — as the malfunction to be medicated, managed, reframed, or breathed through until it quiets enough to be ignored.

But anxiety is not the problem. Anxiety is the signal that a problem exists.

Take the smoke alarm out of a burning building and the building still burns. Take the anxiety out of a life that has accumulated genuine reasons to be anxious and the life continues accumulating those reasons — now without the alarm system that was at least pointing at them. The silence that follows is not peace. It is the specific danger of a fire no longer announced.

What would happen if, instead of managing the anxiety, you followed it? If you allowed the alarm to direct your attention toward the thing it has been going off about — the relationship whose terms are not sustainable, the situation whose costs keep climbing, the internal reality you have been too busy being anxious to actually examine — and addressed the fire rather than the noise?

This does not mean every anxious thought is accurate information. The anxious mind produces false alarms, and distinguishing signal from noise is part of the work. But the pattern of chronic anxiety in a specific context — the relationship, the work environment, the family dynamic that reliably produces it — is almost never purely noise. The alarm keeps going off because the fire keeps burning. Addressing the fire is the only thing that actually makes the alarm stop.

Reflection 43

Chronic pain — physical, emotional, relational — is the body and the heart's long-standing request for something to change. How long have you been ignoring the request?

The research on the relationship between psychological distress and physical illness is now extensive enough to constitute one of the most significant findings in modern medicine. ACEs — adverse childhood experiences — have been documented across multiple large-scale studies to correlate with dramatically increased rates of autoimmune disease, chronic pain conditions, cardiovascular disease, and cancer. The body keeps what the mind refuses to process. Not metaphorically. Measurably. In tissue and inflammatory markers and the specific physiological signatures of a nervous system that has been running in chronic stress activation for long enough that the activation has become the baseline.

The chronic headache. The digestive system that has been unhappy for years. The back that goes out at specific stressful intervals. The immune system that seems to be fighting the wrong things. The specific physical locations where your body holds what your life produces in emotional experience.

These are not separate from the psychological. They are its expression in the only domain the body has available — the physical. When the emotional request goes unanswered long enough, the body submits the same request in its own language. And the body's language tends to be louder and harder to ignore.

This is not to suggest that every physical symptom has a purely psychological origin or that medical care is unnecessary. Medical care is necessary and important. But medical care that treats the symptom without examining the life producing it is incomplete — like mopping the floor without addressing the leak. How long has the water been coming in? What, honestly, would need to change for the request to finally be answered?

Reflection 44

You called it overthinking. It was perception. You called it sensitivity. It was accuracy. You called it too much. It was the truth arriving in the only form available.

The specific labels applied to women's accurate perceptions — overthinking, sensitivity, emotionality, irrationality — function as a disposal mechanism. Take a perception that is correct, label it as a symptom of psychological instability, and the person experiencing it will be more likely to discard it than act on it. The disposal benefits whoever the perception was accurately pointing at.

You called it overthinking because the alternative — accepting that what you were perceiving was real — required a response you were not ready to make. Overthinking can be managed. The truth requires action. So the truth got relabeled into something manageable, filed under personal failing rather than accurate information, and the accurate information got discarded along with it.

You called it sensitivity because the people around you called it that. Because the alternative — their behavior was producing a correct response in you and they were responsible for examining their behavior — was inconvenient for them. Sensitivity is the woman's problem. Insensitivity in the person producing the behavior worthy of response is rarely named in the same conversation.

You called it too much because the environment could not hold what was real, and the thing that cannot be held gets labeled as excess rather than as evidence of the container's inadequacy.

The overthinking was pattern recognition. The sensitivity was emotional intelligence operating at high resolution. The too much was the full truth of your experience arriving at full volume. None of it was the malfunction. All of it was the signal. And the signal was right.

Reflection 45

The breakdown was not a failure. It was the pressure finally becoming greater than the performance could contain.

There is a specific shame attached to breaking down — to the moment when the capacity for maintaining fine runs out and something more honest comes through. The composure fractures. The performance stops. What has been held together through extraordinary effort stops being held and the whole accumulated weight of it lands at once, visibly, often in the most inconvenient possible moment.

And the first response — internal, usually, before anyone else has had time to offer theirs — is failure. I cannot handle this. I am not strong enough. Other people manage without falling apart. Something is wrong with me.

What is actually happening is the opposite of failure. What is happening is that the pressure finally exceeded the infrastructure — that the weight you have been carrying, without adequate support, without honest acknowledgment of what it costs, without the release that appropriate expression of difficulty would have provided, finally became heavier than the performance mechanism could manage.

The breakdown is the body and the psyche refusing, finally, to continue the pretense that everything is fine when everything is not fine. It is the most honest thing that has happened in a long time. It is the thing the performance was preventing — and the performance was preventing it because the truth of it felt too large, too much, too potentially consequential to release in the ordinary flow of daily life.

The breakdown was not the moment you failed. It was the moment the truth finally got through. What you do with it from here determines what it becomes. Responded to honestly, it is the beginning of something that actually works. Covered back over with the performance, it is the preview of the next one.

CHAPTER 10

The Grief Underneath the Suffering

What Has Never Been Properly Mourned

Reflection 46

Underneath the resentment is grief. Underneath the anger is grief. Underneath the numbness is grief. It was always grief.

Grief is the emotion most people will do almost anything to avoid — not because it is the most painful emotion, though it is significant, but because it is the one that requires the most complete surrender. You cannot grieve strategically. You cannot grief-manage your way through it with the same productivity orientation that handles most other difficult feelings. Grief demands that you stop, sit down, and allow the full weight of the loss to be exactly as heavy as it actually is.

Most people prefer almost anything else.

The resentment is more manageable. It is active, directed, energized by a kind of indignation that keeps movement going rather than requiring stillness. The anger is more accessible — it has a target, a logic, a sense of agency that grief does not provide. The numbness is the most effective of all the alternatives because it requires nothing, feels nothing, and asks nothing except the ongoing willingness to remain unavailable to your own interior.

But underneath all of them — underneath the resentment at the people who did not show up for you, underneath the anger at what was taken, underneath the specific flatness of a person who has been feeling nothing for long enough that nothing has become the default — is the grief that was never allowed to be what it was.

The grief for the childhood that should have been different. For the love that was not enough. For the years inside what should have been temporary. For the version of yourself who deserved better than what she received and spent decades trying to make the receiving feel like enough.

That grief is not weakness. It is the honest weight of real loss. And it has been waiting, underneath everything else, for the permission to finally be felt.

Reflection 47

You skipped the grief and went straight to functioning. The grief went nowhere. It became everything else.

The cultural instruction around difficult experience is almost uniformly oriented toward recovery speed. Move through it. Process it. Come out on the other side. Do the work and get back to functioning as quickly as possible, because functioning is what is valued and grief — extended, genuine, non-productive grief — does not have a clear place in lives that are organized around continuous forward motion.

So you functioned. You did the remarkable and exhausting thing of holding yourself together through things that deserved to fall apart, of maintaining the forward motion through losses that deserved stillness, of getting back up before the ground had finished arriving.

The grief that was not felt did not disappear. It does not disappear. It relocated — into the body as the chronic tension that has no specific cause, into the relationships as the resentment that arrives without clear origin, into the creative life as the specific flatness of someone whose emotional range has been compressed to exclude the frequencies that grief requires, into the middle of ordinary moments as the sudden, sourceless sadness that arrives without warning and passes before you have allowed yourself to know what it was actually about.

The grief is in there. It has been in there. It has been operating as everything except what it actually is because everything except grief is more tolerable to the person who learned that grief was not something there was room for.

There is room now. Not comfortable room — grief never inhabits comfortable space. But room enough to finally let it be what it is instead of the thousand other things it has been pretending to be.

Reflection 48

Grieving what you deserved and did not receive is not self-pity. It is the honest acknowledgment of a real loss.

The conflation of grief with self-pity is one of the more damaging confusions in the emotional vocabulary most people inherited. Self-pity is the rumination that keeps you circling the loss without moving through it — the rehearsal of grievance that produces no forward motion and exists primarily as a way of avoiding the more difficult emotions underneath the complaint. Grief is different. Grief is the direct experience of loss — felt fully, without narrative overlay, without the drama of self-pity but with the complete honesty of someone who is allowing the weight to be exactly as heavy as it is.

Grieving that you did not receive the parenting you deserved is not indulgent. The loss was real. Children deserve consistent, attuned, emotionally available caregiving that does not require their self-erasure as the condition of belonging. If you did not receive that, something that was yours by right was not given to you. That is a real loss. It deserves real acknowledgment.

Grieving that years were spent in a relationship that was not what it was presented to be is not weak. The years were real. The investment was real. The hope was real. The gap between what was hoped for and what was actually available is a real gap, and the size of that gap is a real loss, and naming it as loss rather than as personal failure is not self-indulgence. It is accuracy.

You are allowed to grieve what you deserved and did not receive. Not as a permanent residence — grief is not designed to be inhabited indefinitely. But as a necessary stop on the way to wherever you are actually going.

Reflection 49

You cannot heal around the grief. You have to go through it. Every detour you have taken has been the long way around what you needed to feel.

The detours are creative. This needs to be acknowledged. The human capacity for avoiding the thing that most needs to be felt is genuinely impressive in its ingenuity. The busyness that ensures there is never quiet enough for the grief to surface. The intellectualization that understands the loss with great sophistication from a safe cognitive distance. The helping — the orientation of all available energy toward other people's pain so that one's own remains unattended. The new relationship entered before the previous one has been properly mourned, importing the unprocessed grief from the last thing into the emotional territory of the next.

Each detour is understandable. The grief, when it finally arrives in full, is not a comfortable experience. The body often resists it physically — constricting the chest, tightening the throat, producing the specific somatic rebellion of a system that has learned to associate this level of feeling with something intolerable. The mind resists it by generating the story that this is too much, that feeling this fully will be destructive rather than healing, that the better strategy is to continue in the direction away from it.

But every detour extends the journey. The grief is a fixed location between where you are and where you need to go. You can approach it from different angles, at different speeds, with different levels of support. You cannot skip it and arrive at the other side.

The other side is real. People get there — not by avoiding the grief but by moving through it with enough support and enough honest willingness to let it be what it is. The through is not as long as the fear of it suggests. The resistance to it is almost always worse than the experience of it.

Reflection 50

Grief does not mean you lost. It means something was genuinely worth mourning. That is not weakness. That is evidence of a heart that was fully in it.

The people who do not grieve are not the ones who feel less. They are the ones who protected themselves from feeling fully — who held the important things at a distance that made loss manageable but also made love less complete, presence less genuine, the experience of their own life filtered through the gauze of self-protection.

The grief you feel — for the relationship, the childhood, the years, the version of yourself that could not be fully expressed, the love that was not enough, the hope that ran longer than the evidence warranted — that grief is proportionate to the genuineness of your investment. You were not half-present. You were not managing from a safe distance. You were in it, with the full force of your capacity for caring, and the loss is large because what you brought to it was real.

That is not a vulnerability to be corrected. It is the specific quality of a person who knows how to love fully and has paid the price of that capacity in the currency of real loss when the love met circumstances that could not match what she brought to them.

The grief is the measure of your heart. Let it be that. Let it be evidence of something worth grieving rather than proof of some error in how fully you showed up.

The error was never in the fullness. The error, if there was one, was in the direction — in the places that fullness was brought that could not receive it. The capacity itself is not the problem.

It is, in fact, everything you need for what comes next.

CHAPTER 11

The Anger You Were Never Allowed to Have

Reclaiming the Emotion That Was Taken From You

Reflection 51

The anger you suppressed did not disappear. It became your anxiety, your depression, your body's tension, your resentment in quiet moments, your explosion at things too small to justify it.

The transformation of suppressed anger into other psychological and physical presentations is one of the most consistently documented phenomena in clinical psychology and one of the most consistently overlooked in the popular conversation about mental health. Depression, in a significant proportion of cases, is anger turned inward — redirected from its appropriate external target toward the self, who is a safer recipient of the feeling in environments where the external expression has consequences. Anxiety, in many cases, is the energy of unexpressed anger with nowhere to go — a nervous system activated for a response that has been prevented from occurring, the charge with no discharge running continuously through a system not designed for that level of sustained activation.

The chronic tension in the jaw, the shoulders, the neck — the musculature most involved in the physical expression of anger — holding what was never permitted to move. The resentment that appears in the middle of unrelated interactions, disproportionate to the current trigger because it is carrying the accumulated charge of every previous trigger that was suppressed. The explosion at the small thing — the spilled coffee, the minor inconvenience — that carries the emotional force of every large thing that was never allowed to register at its actual size.

The anger went somewhere. It went into your body, your mood, your relationships, your experience of your own mind. It did not become less by being suppressed. It became less legible. Harder to trace to its source. More diffuse in its damage.

Bringing it back into legibility — allowing it to be identified as anger, directed at its actual source, felt as the specific emotion it is rather than the dozen other things it has been masquerading as — is not dangerous. It is the beginning of resolution.

Reflection 52

You were taught that your anger was dangerous. It was dangerous — to the people who needed you to stay quiet.

Examine who taught you this. Whose comfort required your anger to remain suppressed? Whose position of authority depended on your not naming what was happening as something worth being angry about? Whose behavior would have required examination or change if you had been permitted to respond to it with the honest emotional response it warranted?

The instruction not to be angry was almost never about you. It was not delivered because your anger was genuinely destructive or because expressing it would have produced harm. It was delivered because your anger — honest, accurately directed, proportionate to what produced it — was inconvenient. It was pointing at something that the person who needed you to suppress it did not want pointed at.

You received the instruction and internalized it as truth about yourself. Your anger is too much. Your anger is inappropriate. Your anger means something is wrong with you rather than with what produced it. Your anger is a symptom of your instability rather than an accurate response to someone else's behavior.

This is how an entire generation of women learned to suppress the emotion most directly connected to the experience of violation. Not through a single explicit instruction but through the consistent environmental message that their anger made things difficult, made them difficult, was somehow both their responsibility to manage and evidence against them.

Your anger was not dangerous to you. It was dangerous to the people it was accurately directed at. And the people it was accurately directed at were the ones with the power to teach you that dangerous meant bad rather than informative.

Reflection 53

Anger at what genuinely wronged you is not a character flaw. It is the correct emotional response to an actual violation.

The capacity for anger is not a design defect in human emotional architecture. It is a specifically designed response to a specific category of experience — the experience of violation, of having something taken or damaged or disregarded that was rightfully yours to protect. Anger, in its healthy form, is the emotion that says this was wrong and I know it was wrong and I am not going to pretend otherwise. It is the emotional correlate of a clear-eyed assessment that a line was crossed.

In healthy functioning, anger is specific, temporary, directed at its actual source, and motivates response rather than rumination. It arrives, it says its thing, it points at what needs to be addressed, and it resolves when the situation has been adequately responded to or when the person has genuinely accepted what cannot be changed and grieved accordingly.

The anger that lingers indefinitely, that has no resolution, that keeps cycling without diminishing — that is suppressed anger that was never allowed to complete its arc. The problem with that anger is not the anger itself but the suppression that prevented it from doing what it was designed to do.

You are allowed to be angry about what was done to you. The anger does not make you bitter or damaged or someone who cannot let go. The anger that has nowhere to go becomes those things. The anger that is finally acknowledged, directed accurately, and allowed to inform your understanding of what you deserve — that anger becomes clarity. And clarity is exactly what you need.

Reflection 54

The woman who is never angry has not transcended anger. She has buried it under something that is slowly poisoning the well.

The transcendence narrative around anger — the idea that the spiritually or psychologically evolved woman has moved beyond anger, that her peacefulness is evidence of growth rather than suppression — has caused significant harm to women who absorbed it and applied it to the project of their own ongoing self-management.

Real equanimity — the genuine, lived, unperformed peacefulness of a person who has processed what happened to them and made their peace with it — is possible and it is beautiful and it is worth working toward. It does not look like the absence of anger at violations. It looks like anger that completes its arc rather than getting suppressed — that arrives, informs, motivates the appropriate response, and resolves because it was allowed to do its work.

What the never-angry woman has is not this. What she has is a sophisticated suppression system operating in real time, converting the anger into acceptable forms as fast as it arrives. Sweetness. Accommodation. The specific pleasantness of someone who has decided that expressing anything that might disturb the atmosphere is not worth the cost.

The cost of the suppression is invisible from the outside and corrosive from the inside. The well that it poisons is not first the relationships or the circumstances. It is the woman herself — her vitality, her capacity for genuine feeling across the full range, her relationship with her own perceptions and their validity.

The not-angry woman is not healed. She is managed. And management, however sophisticated, is not the same as freedom.

Reflection 55

Your anger has information. Before you release it, receive it. It knows something you have been trying not to know.

Anger is not primarily an emotion to be expressed. It is primarily an emotion to be read. Before the expression — before deciding what to do with it or whether and how to communicate it — the anger deserves to be received as the information it is carrying. What specifically happened that produced this response? What was violated? What does the intensity of the anger indicate about the significance of the violation? What has the anger been trying to direct your attention toward that the suppression has been successfully keeping out of focus?

The anger at the relationship that has not been honoring your worth has been pointing at the relationship's inadequacy for longer than you have been willing to look in that direction. The anger at the dynamic that keeps reproducing itself has been identifying the dynamic as something that needs to change for longer than you have been willing to accept that it probably will not change on its own. The anger at yourself — the specific, relentless, directed-inward anger that has been presenting as self-criticism and inadequacy — is almost always the externally directed anger that was too risky to express and got turned around on the safer target.

Receive the anger before you release it. Let it be a conversation rather than just a discharge. Ask it what it is actually about — not the surface event that triggered it but the underlying reality it has been pointing at. The anger knows. It has known for a long time. It has been trying, through the anxiety and the depression and the resentment and the explosion at small things, to tell you what it knows.

Let it tell you. Finally, directly, without immediately suppressing the message. The information it is carrying is something you need to have.

***

"She had spent so many years turning her pain into performance, her anger into accommodation, her grief into functioning, that when someone finally asked her how she was doing — really doing — she sat with the question for a long time before she could answer. Not because she did not know. Because she was not yet sure she was allowed to say."

PART FOUR: WHAT HEALING ACTUALLY REQUIRES

The Honest, Uncomfortable, Necessary Work of Stopping the Betrayal

CHAPTER 12

Healing Is Not What They Showed You

Dismantling the Fantasy of Recovery and Replacing It With the Reality

---

Reflection 56

Healing is not the return to who you were before the wound. That person does not exist anymore. Healing is becoming someone who has integrated what happened and is no longer governed by it.

The before-and-after framework for healing is one of the most quietly damaging stories we tell about recovery. It suggests a destination that does not exist — a return to a self that predates the damage, intact and restored, the wound erased rather than incorporated. People wait for this return. They measure their progress by how close they are to getting back to the person they were before, and when that person does not reappear, they conclude that the healing has failed.

The person you were before the wound was shaped by everything that preceded the wound. She was not the final version. She was an earlier one, and the wound — like everything that came before it — was part of the process of becoming who you are now and who you are still in the process of becoming. You cannot return to her any more than you can return to yourself at fifteen. The timeline does not run backward.

What healing actually produces is not restoration. It is integration — the genuine incorporation of what happened into a self that is larger than the wound rather than organized around it. The integrated person carries the mark of what happened the way a healed bone carries the mark of the break — not invisible, not pretended away, but incorporated into a structure that is often stronger at the site of the old fracture than it would have been without it.

She does not forget. She does not arrive at the point where the wound is no longer part of her history. She arrives at the point where the wound is no longer the primary organizing principle of her present — where it has taken its proper place in the full, complicated, genuinely hers story of her life rather than occupying the center of it.

That is not a lesser version of healed. That is the only version that is actually available. And it is more interesting, more genuinely earned, more fully alive than the fantasy of return.

Reflection 57

Healing is not linear. It is not a before and after. It is the same territory walked repeatedly, each time with slightly better equipment.

The linear model of healing — you begin, you progress, you arrive — is a story borrowed from physical injury, where the wound closes and the tissue regenerates in a sequence that roughly follows a predictable timeline. Psychological healing does not follow this model, and the expectation that it should is responsible for enormous amounts of unnecessary shame in people who are genuinely doing the work.

You will revisit the same material repeatedly. Not because the previous visit failed — because psychological material has layers, and what is accessible in the first visit is only what can be held with the resources available at that time. As the resources develop, deeper layers become accessible. The revisiting is not regression. It is descent — the same territory entered more deeply because you are now equipped to go further than before.

The person who has been in genuine healing work for three years visits the childhood wound differently than she did in the first year — with more compassion, more nuance, more ability to hold the complexity without needing it to resolve into a simple narrative. The visit feels familiar because the territory is familiar. It is different because she is.

The setback that looks like losing ground is almost always the beginning of the next layer. The return of old feelings after a period of what felt like resolution is not evidence that the resolution was false. It is the announcement that there is more — that the work went far enough to produce the stability necessary to hold what comes next.

Trust the spiral. The same territory walked with better equipment is not the same experience. It is the next one.

Reflection 58

Some days healing looks like a breakthrough. More days it looks like doing the ordinary thing without the old weight. Both count.

The breakthroughs get the attention. The session that cracked something open. The conversation that shifted something that had been immovable. The moment of clarity that reorganized the entire story into something that finally made coherent sense. These moments are real and they matter and they deserve acknowledgment.

But they are not where most of healing lives. Most of healing lives in the Tuesday afternoon when you respond to a minor frustration without the disproportionate reaction that would have arrived six months ago. In the conversation where you say the thing you would have previously swallowed and discover that the world remains intact. In the night you sleep without the particular anxiety that used to occupy the three-to-five space of your sleep architecture. In the moment you catch the old pattern activating and make a different choice — not dramatically, not with any particular fanfare, just differently.

These moments do not feel like healing. They feel like ordinary life. That is exactly what they are — and ordinary life lived without the old weight is the most concrete available evidence that something has actually changed.

The metric for healing is not the intensity of the insight. It is the quality of the ordinary day. The baseline emotional texture of a Tuesday. The specific presence or absence of the chronic low-level suffering that became so normalized you stopped registering it as suffering.

Track the ordinary days. The progress is in them, accumulated quietly and consistently, building the new baseline that eventually becomes the normal you did not know was possible.

Reflection 59

You will heal in the relationships that required you to break. You will also heal in the ones that were present when you did. Both are part of the same process.

The wound arrived in relationship. The earliest ones — the attachment relationships that installed the templates for love and safety and worth — were relational before they were anything else. The patterns that developed in response to those relationships were relational adaptations. The betrayal of self that accumulated across years happened in the context of relationships that rewarded it.

Healing that does not eventually include relationship is incomplete — not because solo work lacks value, but because the nervous system that was shaped in relationship will not fully update without new relational experience to update it against. You can understand the attachment wound completely in therapy and still find it running in your body the moment a specific kind of intimacy arrives. The understanding is necessary. It is not sufficient.

Some healing happens in the difficult relationships — the ones that activated the wound sharply enough to make it impossible to continue ignoring. These relationships, painful as they were, performed the service of making what was invisible impossible to avoid. The person who triggered the pattern most reliably was often the one who made the pattern undeniable.

Some healing happens in the safe relationships — the ones that were present in the aftermath, that held you without requiring your performance, that showed you through the direct experience of being genuinely witnessed what consistent care and genuine regard actually feel like in the body. These are the relationships that begin to update the template — not through instruction but through the irreplaceable medium of lived experience.

Both kinds of relationship are part of the process. Neither alone is the whole.

Reflection 60

The timeline is yours. Not your family's. Not your therapist's. Not the person who healed faster and keeps telling you about it.

The comparison of healing timelines is one of the more counterproductive activities available to a person in the process of recovery, and it is nearly impossible to avoid in a culture where healing has become, in some spaces, a performance with visible metrics and public milestones. Someone else's breakthrough becomes a standard. Someone else's timeline becomes a measure of your own pace. Someone else's readiness to move on becomes evidence that you are not moving fast enough.

Your timeline is determined by factors that are entirely specific to you — the depth of the original wound, the resources available during the period when the damage was occurring, the quality of support available since, the specific nature of the patterns that developed, the degree to which the patterns have been reinforced across years of subsequent experience. None of these factors are the same as the factors that governed someone else's timeline. The comparison is therefore meaningless as a measure of progress and harmful as an emotional experience.

Your family's timeline for your healing is based on their comfort with your process rather than any accurate assessment of what your process requires. Their readiness for you to be done is not information about where you actually are. Your therapist's timeline, if it exists, is a clinical approximation that may or may not correspond to the specific pace of your particular healing — and a good therapist knows this and does not impose it.

The pace at which genuine healing occurs is the pace at which it can be genuinely integrated. Faster than that is not healing. It is the performance of healing — which is indistinguishable from the original performance of fine and produces similar long-term results.

Take the time the work actually requires. That is the only timeline that produces something real.

CHAPTER 13

What You Have to Be Willing to Lose

The Specific Surrenders That Genuine Healing Requires

Reflection 61

You will have to lose the identity you built around the suffering. That identity is familiar. Losing it will feel like losing yourself. It is the opposite.

The identity constructed around suffering is one of the most stable and most thoroughly occupied structures in a human life. It is built from genuine experience, reinforced across years of consistent inhabitation, and connected to the relationships, the roles, the sense of self and purpose that developed inside it. It is not a thin or superficial thing. It is the entire house.

Who are you without the wound as your organizing center? Who are you when you are not the survivor, the one who endures, the person who carries what others cannot? Who are you when the suffering is no longer the context within which your identity makes sense?

These are not rhetorical questions. They are the actual disorientation of someone whose house is being demolished. And they produce, in many people at this stage of healing, a pull back toward the wound — not because the wound is desirable but because the identity it houses is the only self that has been fully inhabited. The unfamiliar self on the other side of the healing has not yet been built out. It exists as possibility rather than lived experience, and possibility is a thin place to stand when what you are leaving is the only solid ground you have known.

You lose the suffering-identity not by deciding to abandon it but by gradually building something else — by accumulating enough experience of the non-suffering self that it develops enough substance to be habitable. The loss is real. The grief for it is legitimate. And what replaces it is not nothing. It is the self that was always underneath the wound, waiting for the wound to stop requiring all the available real estate.

That self is more interesting than the wound. She has been waiting long enough.

Reflection 62

You will have to lose the relationships that required your pain to function. Some of them love you. Love is not sufficient if it needs you broken to stay.

This is the hardest loss in the entire catalog of what healing requires, and naming it plainly is an act of care rather than cruelty. Because it needs to be named — because the relationships that are organized around your suffering will not simply dissolve as you heal without anyone having to acknowledge what is happening.

Some of the people who love you have built their relationship with you inside the specific dynamic of your wound. Not from malice — most of the time. From their own wounds, their own needs, the specific way that your suffering intersected with their relational patterns to produce a dynamic that worked for both of you in the specific way that unhealthy dynamics work — by providing each person with the familiar emotional landscape they were calibrated for.

The relationship that needed you to need saving. The connection that functioned primarily around your difficulty and had no established way of being together outside of it. The friendship that was organized around your mutual suffering and that will have nothing in common with you when the suffering is no longer the shared language.

These are real losses. The love in them, where it exists, is real. And love — genuine, warmly felt, historically significant love — is not sufficient to make a relationship sustainable if the relationship's structure requires your ongoing pain as its operating condition.

You do not have to end them dramatically. Some of them will shift as you shift — finding a new shape that can hold the changed version of you. Some will not, and the ending will come from the natural dissolution of a dynamic whose terms no longer apply. Let both happen. Grieve both honestly. Neither loss means you were wrong to leave the suffering behind.

Reflection 63

You will have to lose the story that what happened to you defined you. It shaped you. It does not own you.

The defining story is subtler than it appears. It does not always present as victimhood or as the explicit narrative of damage. Sometimes it presents as the explanation for everything — the origin story that gets deployed to account for every difficulty, every pattern, every response that needs context. The wound becomes the through-line of the life, the lens through which every subsequent experience is understood.

This is not without value in the early stages of healing. Understanding how the wound shaped the patterns — making the invisible visible, providing context for responses that had previously seemed inexplicable — is genuinely important work. The causal connection between early experience and current functioning is real and worth understanding.

The point where the story shifts from useful to limiting is the point where it stops being the explanation for patterns you are working to change and becomes the permanent account of who you are. When the wound is no longer the origin story but the identity story — when you are the person this happened to rather than the person who is building something in response to what happened — the story has shifted from clarifying to constraining.

What happened to you is real. The shaping it did is real. Neither of these facts makes what happened the final word on who you are or what your life can be. The shaping produced a self that has navigated extraordinary things and is still standing and is still capable of change and growth and a life that is genuinely and specifically hers.

That self is not defined by her wound. She is enlarged by having survived it and done the work of integrating it.

Reflection 64

You will have to lose the hope that the person who hurt you will eventually acknowledge it. The acknowledgment you need cannot come from them. Build it from inside.

The waiting for acknowledgment is one of the most consuming and most costly of the places where healing stalls. Not because the desire for it is unreasonable — the desire for the person who caused harm to name what they did, to see the impact, to offer the genuine accountability that would allow the wound to finally have a witness — is one of the most human desires available. The wish to be seen in the hurt, by the person whose actions produced it, is not pathological. It is the original need for repair that goes unmet in every significant wound.

The problem is the dependency. When the healing waits on the acknowledgment — when the ability to move forward is structurally dependent on receiving something from someone who has, in most cases, demonstrated through their behavior that the acknowledgment is not forthcoming — the healing is in the hands of the person who caused the damage. And the person who caused the damage is almost never the person most motivated to provide what is needed for the person they damaged to recover.

The acknowledgment you actually need — the deep, cellular-level recognition that what happened to you was real, was wrong, was not what you deserved, and does not reflect on your worth — cannot be provided from outside at that depth. It can be offered from outside. Therapy offers versions of it. Honest relationships offer versions of it. But the version that actually heals is the one you build yourself, from inside, through the accumulated experience of treating yourself as someone whose experience of what happened matters enough to be taken seriously.

Stop waiting for the acknowledgment from the source. Become the witness you needed. That is not settling. That is the most direct available route to the freedom you are waiting for their acknowledgment to provide.

Reflection 65

Everything you lose in the process of healing was either genuinely yours and will return in a different form, or it was never genuinely yours. Either way, the losing is necessary.

This reflection is the one to return to when the losses feel like too much — when the relationships are changing and the identity is dissolving and the stories are being relinquished and the hope for external acknowledgment is being released and everything that was stable in the old life seems to be in motion at once.

What is genuinely yours cannot ultimately be taken by healing. The capacity for love — that remains. The intelligence and the sensitivity and the specific qualities that were present before the wound and have persisted through it — those remain and in many cases are amplified by the process of honest examination rather than diminished by it. The relationships that are genuinely based in mutual regard and that can survive your growth — those remain, often deepened by the changes rather than threatened by them.

What does not survive the healing was not built on solid ground. The relationships organized around your wound. The identity constructed from your suffering. The stories that required your smallness to hold together. The hope that was manufacturing basis for itself in the absence of actual evidence. These do not survive because they were not, ultimately, yours — they were the specific constructions of a life organized around pain, and a life no longer organized around pain has no architecture for them.

The losing is not punishment. It is the natural consequence of becoming someone for whom the old structures no longer fit. The things that are actually yours will find their way back in forms appropriate to who you are becoming. The things that do not come back were keeping you from exactly this.

Let them go. Not easily, not without grief, not with any pretense that the losing is not real. But let them go.

CHAPTER 14

The Work That Cannot Be Skipped

Accountability, Honesty, and the Parts of Healing Most People Try to Go Around

---

Reflection 66

You cannot think your way to healed. The work lives below the level of insight.

The most common version of healing avoidance in psychologically sophisticated people is the accumulation of insight without behavioral change. It is entirely possible — common, in fact — to build a comprehensive, nuanced, clinically accurate understanding of your own wound while remaining completely inside the patterns the wound produced. The understanding is real. The change is not happening. The gap between them is the most frustrating place in healing to be, because from the inside it looks like doing the work and from the outside it looks like doing the work and from the perspective of actual change, it is the appearance of doing the work without the substance of it.

Insight lives in the cortex. The patterns being addressed live in the subcortex — in the amygdala, the brainstem, the body, the nervous system's operating logic that predates language and is not accessible to the thinking brain in any direct way. Understanding the pattern at the cortical level does not update it at the subcortical level. The nervous system does not respond to explanation. It responds to experience.

The work that actually changes the pattern is not more understanding. It is new behavior — the body doing the different thing, the nervous system experiencing a different outcome, the lived evidence accumulating that what happens when you act differently is survivable and eventually preferable. This requires doing uncomfortable things before they feel comfortable, which is the part that understanding consistently fails to produce on its own.

The insight is the necessary starting point. It is not the destination. The destination is in what you do with your body and your choices in the moments when the pattern activates and the old behavior is what every trained impulse is pointing toward.

Reflection 67

Understanding why you are the way you are is not the same as changing it. Understanding is the map. The territory requires your body, your behavior, and your daily choices.

Maps are extraordinary tools. They compress complex terrain into navigable information. They allow you to understand the relationship between where you are and where you are going without having to physically traverse every inch of the ground between them. For planning, for orientation, for the development of strategy — maps are indispensable.

You cannot live in a map. The map of your psychology — the understanding of how the wound formed and what adaptations developed and what patterns those adaptations produced and why those patterns have persisted — is genuinely useful information. It is not a substitute for the actual journey.

The actual journey requires the body. The nervous system that keeps choosing the familiar has to accumulate enough direct experience of choosing differently to begin updating its operating logic. The muscles that have been holding chronic tension have to practice releasing it, repeatedly, until release becomes available. The voice that was trained to silence itself has to practice speaking, in small moments first and then in larger ones, until speaking feels like less of an emergency.

The daily choices are the territory. Not the dramatic choices — not the ones that come with obvious stakes and clear decision points. The ordinary daily choices. The moment of choosing rest over performance. The moment of speaking instead of swallowing. The moment of staying in the unfamiliar peace instead of manufacturing familiar chaos. These moments are where the map either becomes a journey or remains a document.

Reflection 68

At some point you have to stop explaining the wound and start making different choices in spite of it.

The wound deserves explanation. The context of how the patterns formed, the intelligence of the adaptations, the genuine difficulty of what was survived — all of this deserves honest articulation and genuine compassion. The work of understanding is real and necessary and should not be rushed.

And at some point it becomes the thing that keeps you in place.

The explanation that was once the beginning of self-understanding becomes the permanent account that makes change feel optional rather than possible. The context that was once the antidote to shame becomes the reason that new choices cannot yet be made. The story of the wound becomes the justification for the wound's ongoing governance of behavior — not because the story is false, but because the story has been substituted for the work of actually doing something different.

This shift is subtle and it is common and it is worth naming plainly because the people most likely to be reading this are often the most sophisticated explainers of their own psychology. The sophistication is real. The insight is genuine. And it has become, at some inflection point that is worth honestly locating, the thing that makes the actual behavioral change feel less urgent than it is.

You are allowed to have the wound and make different choices in spite of it. The two things are not in conflict. The different choice does not deny the wound. It simply refuses to let the wound have the final word about what is available to you now.

That refusal is the work. Not the explanation of why the refusal is difficult. The refusal itself.

Reflection 69

The part of the healing work you keep avoiding is almost certainly the part where the most significant change is waiting.

The avoidance is not random. It is directed, consistently and with impressive precision, toward exactly the material that would produce the most change if engaged. This is not a coincidence. The psyche avoids what threatens its current structure, and what most threatens the current structure is what would most significantly alter it.

The letters never written to the people who caused harm. Not to send — to feel the full weight of what happened and what it cost, without the protective distance of clinical understanding. The grief that has been scheduled for later indefinitely. The relationship conversation that has been prepared for in therapy for eight months without being had. The physical practice — the somatic work, the body-based approach — that keeps being meant to start next week.

The avoidance is intelligent. What is being avoided is genuinely threatening to the current equilibrium, and the current equilibrium, however costly, is at least known. What waits on the other side of the avoided material is unknown, and unknown activates the same threat response as danger regardless of whether the unknown is actually dangerous.

The thing you keep not doing is the next thing. Not because avoiding it has made it smaller — avoided material typically grows rather than diminishes — but because engaging it is what the avoidance has been preventing, and the avoidance has been preventing it because something in you knows it will matter.

Name the avoidance specifically. Not the general category — not I avoid vulnerability or I avoid grief. The specific thing. The specific undone work. Then ask what would have to be true for you to do it this week.

Reflection 70

You get to keep being hurt by what happened. You do not get to keep using it as the reason you cannot move.

These two things are not in conflict, and holding both simultaneously is the exact balance that genuine healing requires. The hurt is permanent in the sense that what happened happened and left a mark and the mark is real. The hurt is not permanent in the sense of having the right to govern your choices indefinitely regardless of the work you have done and the resources you have built.

Being hurt by what happened is not weakness. It is not insufficient healing. It is the accurate ongoing response of a person to whom something genuinely damaging occurred. The healing is not the absence of hurt. It is the presence of a self who can be hurt without being stopped — who carries the reality of what happened without being organized around it, who feels the grief when it arrives without the grief determining what is available to her.

The wound as reason — the ongoing deployment of what happened as the explanation for why different choices cannot yet be made, why the relationship cannot be risked, why the work cannot begin, why the life that might be available remains out of reach — that is the part that healing is asking you to examine. Not because the wound is not real. Because the wound has been doing double duty as both the mark of what happened and the limit of what is possible, and those are two different things.

The mark stays. The limit does not have to.

CHAPTER 15

Asking for Help Without Calling It Weakness

The Courage Required to Stop Carrying Everything Alone

Reflection 71

The most self-sufficient women are often the most profoundly lonely. The self-sufficiency was never the goal. It was the survival strategy.

Somewhere between needing too much — which produced consequences too painful to repeat — and asking for nothing, there was a calculation made. The calculation was rational. The math was clear enough from the available evidence: needing things from people is dangerous in the specific way that it makes you dependent on their response, and their response has been unreliable in ways that cost you, and the cost of unreliable response is greater than the cost of simply not needing.

So the self-sufficiency was installed. The system for managing everything internally was constructed and refined over years until it operated with the efficiency of something that has been practiced so long it no longer requires conscious attention. And it worked, in the specific sense that it prevented the particular pain of reaching toward someone and having the reaching go unanswered.

What it did not prevent was the loneliness that is structural to a life where the reaching has been removed from the architecture. You can be surrounded by people and profoundly alone if the version of you that is present with them is the self-sufficient one — capable and competent and not requiring anything — while the version of you that actually needs something waits somewhere private that nobody is ever invited into.

The loneliness is the cost of the strategy. It was a cost worth paying when the alternative was the pain of unmet need in relationships that were unreliable. It is a cost worth re-examining now, when the alternative is relationships that might actually be capable of meeting what the self-sufficient version has been preventing anyone from knowing you need.

Reflection 72

Asking for help is not the admission of inadequacy. It is the acknowledgment of reality — that you are human and humans are not built to carry everything alone.

The belief that asking for help reveals inadequacy was installed in an environment where need was either treated as inconvenient or used against you. Where the expression of need produced either withdrawal — the specific abandonment of someone whose availability was contingent on your not requiring anything — or ammunition. Where what you needed was noted and later deployed as evidence of your insufficiency at the precise moment when that evidence would cause the most damage.

In that environment, self-sufficiency was not a character trait. It was a rational protective response to a documented pattern of outcomes. Need equals vulnerability. Vulnerability equals exposure. Exposure equals harm. Therefore: eliminate need. Or at least eliminate its expression, which to the nervous system that learned this early amounts to the same thing.

The protection was appropriate then. In the relationships and circumstances of your current life, it is worth examining which of them operate on the same principles that installed the strategy in the first place. Some do. Those relationships deserve the self-sufficiency, which in that context is still the accurate response to demonstrated reality.

Many do not. Many of the people in your current life have not demonstrated the pattern the strategy was installed to protect against. They have demonstrated something different — the capacity for genuine response, the willingness to hold what you offer them, the specific care of someone who wants to know what you actually need rather than requiring you to perform needlessness as the condition of belonging.

Asking them is not the repetition of the original dangerous act. It is the update — the new behavior tried in new conditions, which is the only way the nervous system ever learns that new conditions exist.

Reflection 73

The therapist, the trusted friend, the support group, the book that finally names it — these are not crutches. They are the resources that were always supposed to be available to you and were not.

The framing of external support as weakness rather than as appropriate resource is cultural, gendered, and enormously costly. The woman who goes to therapy is working on herself in a way that is effortful and courageous and indicative of genuine commitment to change. The cultural reflex that frames the same woman as someone who cannot handle things on her own is not a neutral observation about her capacity. It is a preference — for the version of her that manages everything internally and makes no demands on the system around her.

The resources were always supposed to be available. The consistent, attuned, emotionally present caregiving that builds secure attachment. The family system that could hold your full emotional range without requiring you to manage yourself for everyone else's comfort. The community that witnessed difficulty without prescribing its resolution or its timeline. The relationships that asked what you needed rather than assuming your needs were the category least worth addressing.

If those resources were not available — if you grew up in an environment where the internal management system was installed because the external resources were insufficient or absent or actively harmful — then the therapy and the trusted friendship and the book that names what happened are not supplementing adequate support. They are providing the first adequate support you have had access to.

Receiving them is not weakness. It is the correction of a deficit that was never your fault to have in the first place.

Reflection 74

You spent years being strong for everyone else. Be willing to be held for once. Let someone else carry something.

The woman who is always the holder, the carrier, the one who absorbs and manages and supports and stabilizes everyone else in her orbit — she is performing an extraordinary service to the people around her. She is also depriving both herself and those people of something important.

She is depriving herself of the specific relief of being held — of the experience of bringing something real to another person and having it received with the genuine care and genuine competence that she has been providing to everyone else. The experience of not having to manage your own weight for a moment. Of being the one in the chair rather than the one behind it. Of being genuinely permitted to be wherever you actually are rather than wherever your functioning requires you to appear.

She is also depriving the people who would hold her, if allowed, of the experience of genuine reciprocity. The relationships where one person does all the carrying and the other does all the being-carried are not intimate relationships. They are service relationships — and the service provider and the service recipient are both diminished by the arrangement, however comfortable it is for the person not doing the carrying.

The people who genuinely love you want to hold something for you. Not because they are performing caregiving but because reciprocity is how genuine connection actually works — how two people become genuinely known to each other rather than known in the curated, high-functioning, I-have-everything-handled version that never lets the other person in.

Put something down. Let someone else carry it. Not because you cannot — you have proved beyond any reasonable doubt that you can carry extraordinary things. Because you were never supposed to carry them alone.

Reflection 75

The woman who cannot receive care cannot truly give it. Let yourself be cared for. It is not a contradiction of your strength. It is the proof of it.

Receiving care requires vulnerability. The vulnerability of being seen in need. The vulnerability of allowing someone else to be capable of something in your direction when you have spent years being the capable one. The vulnerability of not knowing, in advance, whether what you offer when you ask for something will be received with the warmth you need or whether the old pattern will repeat and the offering will produce the original consequence.

This is why the self-sufficient woman cannot simply decide to receive care and find it suddenly available to her emotional system. The decision is not the barrier. The vulnerability is. And the vulnerability requires — requires, not just recommends — the experience of having it produce safety rather than the consequences that installed the self-sufficiency in the first place.

That experience comes from trying. From the small, initial, carefully chosen reaching toward people who have demonstrated enough reliability to make the risk calculable. From allowing the help in the low-stakes moment before the high-stakes one. From building, through gradual exposure to the experience of safe receiving, the evidence that this is possible — that the old pattern is not the only pattern available, that need expressed in safe relationship produces something different from what it produced in the relationship where the self-sufficiency was installed.

And what happens to the quality of the giving when the receiving becomes possible? It expands. Because genuine giving — the kind that comes from genuine fullness rather than from the performance of generosity — requires that the giver also be given to. The woman who cannot be filled cannot give from fullness. She gives from depletion, and depletion eventually runs out.

Fill up. Receive. Let someone be capable in your direction for once.

Your giving will be better for it. And you — the woman who has been giving everything to everyone for longer than your body can account for — you deserve to receive something genuinely good.

***

"She had held everyone else up for so long that when someone finally offered to hold her, she did not know what to do with her hands. She stood there with them empty, which was the most honest they had been in years."

PART FIVE: THE PATTERNS THAT KEEP YOU STUCK

Breaking the Cycles That Masquerade as Comfort

CHAPTER 16

The Repetition Compulsion — Why You Keep Recreating the Wound

Understanding the Unconscious Drive to Repeat What Was Never Resolved

Reflection 76

You did not return to the same kind of person, the same dynamic, the same pain because you are broken. You returned because unresolved things seek resolution — even in the wrong places.

Freud called it the repetition compulsion. He noticed it in his patients with a consistency that eventually made the pattern undeniable — that people did not simply remember their traumatic experiences. They re-enacted them. They unconsciously constructed situations that replicated the original wound, populated those situations with people who played the familiar roles, and moved through the dynamic with the specific emotional knowledge of someone who had been here before — because they had. Many times. In slightly different costumes.

The compulsion is not pathological in the sense of indicating something fundamentally wrong with the person experiencing it. It is the psyche's persistent attempt to do something it was not able to do the first time — to get the different ending, the repair, the resolution that the original experience denied. The child who was abandoned seeks relationships where the attachment is insecure because the insecure attachment is the familiar context and the familiar context is where the nervous system believes resolution might finally be achieved. If this person stays this time, if this dynamic resolves differently, the original wound gets retroactively repaired.

It does not work that way. The resolution of the original wound cannot be achieved by repeating its structure in new relationships. The new relationship is not the original one. The new person cannot provide the healing that the original wound requires because they are not the source of the wound. They are simply the most recent recipient of the projection of it.

Understanding this removes the self-blame from the pattern without removing the responsibility for changing it. You were not seeking pain. You were seeking resolution. The search was intelligent and the method was wrong, and knowing the difference is what makes it possible to redirect the search toward something that can actually deliver what it has been looking for.

Reflection 77

The pattern is not punishment. It is the wound looking for the ending it never got.

The ending the wound needs is not available in the repetition of its own structure. This is the tragedy and the mechanism of the repetition compulsion simultaneously — the wound seeks resolution by recreating the conditions of its origin, and the conditions of its origin are precisely the conditions that prevent the resolution the wound is seeking.

The parent who was emotionally unavailable cannot be replaced by an emotionally unavailable partner who finally becomes available. The relationship will replicate the structure but not resolve the original experience, because the original experience belongs to a specific developmental period, involved a specific person with a specific irreplaceable role, and required a specific response that only that person, in that context, could have provided and did not.

What the wound actually needs is not the repetition with a better ending. It is the acknowledgment that the original ending was real and insufficient, the grief for what was not received, and the building of a self who can exist fully and love genuinely without requiring the original deficit to be retroactively corrected by a relationship that was not there for the original experience.

This is why the ending has never arrived in the repetition. Not because the people were wrong, though sometimes they were. Not because you chose badly, though sometimes the pattern did direct you toward people who replicated the wound most precisely. But because the repetition was always aimed at the wrong target. The wound is in the past. Its resolution is in the present — in the work, in the honest grief, in the building of internal resource that makes external correction no longer necessary.

The pattern was not punishing you. It was trying to heal you through the only mechanism it knew. The mechanism was wrong. The need it was serving was real.

Reflection 78

Until the original wound is addressed, you will keep finding new containers for the same pain. Different person. Same dynamic. Same eventual destruction. Same confusion about why this keeps happening.

The containers change with impressive reliability. The relationship ends and the pattern waits a respectful period before appearing in the next one. Sometimes it appears immediately — the rebound that replicates the previous dynamic so precisely it might be the same relationship wearing different features. Sometimes it takes longer, years even, during which the pattern may be genuinely dormant or may simply be less visible because the circumstances that activate it most clearly are not yet present.

And then the new container arrives. The new person. The new situation. And the pattern, which has not gone anywhere, which has simply been waiting for the relevant environmental conditions to reassemble, resumes exactly where it left off.

The containers being new is not the same as the content being new. You can move cities, change jobs, end the relationship, start therapy, read every book in the relevant section of the bookstore, and find the pattern waiting for you in the next relationship because the pattern is not in the relationship. It is in you — in the nervous system's operating logic, in the unconscious template for what intimate experience feels like, in the specific attunement to the emotional signature of the original wound that makes certain people feel immediately familiar in a way that has nothing to do with their actual character.

The container is not the problem. New containers will not solve it. The original wound addressed — not managed, not understood from a comfortable distance, but genuinely entered and processed with adequate support — is what changes the content. And changed content finds genuinely different containers because it is no longer using the familiar-pain template to select them.

Reflection 79

Recognition is not the same as resolution. You can see the pattern clearly and still be pulled by it. The pull is physiological. Changing it requires more than awareness.

This is the point where most psychologically sophisticated people stall, and the stalling produces a specific and demoralizing confusion — the belief that seeing the pattern clearly should be sufficient to break it, and that continuing to be pulled by it despite clear sight is evidence of a deeper dysfunction than the pattern itself.

The confusion arises from the mistaken model of how patterns work. If the pattern were primarily a cognitive phenomenon — a belief system operating at the level of conscious thought — then seeing it clearly would indeed be substantially effective. Cognitive patterns are responsive to cognitive intervention. Seeing them clearly changes the quality of engagement with them in meaningful ways.

The repetition compulsion is not primarily cognitive. It is physiological — encoded in the nervous system's operating logic, in the body's learned response to specific emotional stimuli, in the subcortical pattern-recognition system that processes threat and familiarity faster than conscious thought and that does not receive the cortical awareness as information relevant to its function.

The amygdala does not read the journal. The nervous system does not attend the therapy session in the sense of updating its operating logic based on what was discussed there. The update happens in the body, through new experience, through the repeated direct encounter with a different outcome when the old trigger arrives. Through the nervous system learning, slowly and through accumulation rather than insight, that the familiar pattern is no longer the only available response.

Awareness is the necessary starting point. The necessary continuation is the specific, repeated, behavioral practice of doing something different when the pull arrives — not because the pull has disappeared but because you have developed enough of a pause between the pull and the response to make a different choice in that pause.

Reflection 80

The cycle breaks not when you understand it but when the work you have done makes the familiar pain genuinely less compelling than the unfamiliar peace.

The breaking point is not intellectual. It is not the moment of finally, completely understanding the pattern — the pattern has probably been understood for some time before the cycle actually breaks. The breaking point is experiential. It is the specific moment when the pull toward the familiar painful thing is met by enough internal resource — enough experience of something different, enough accumulated evidence that the unfamiliar is survivable, enough genuine self-regard to make the cost of the familiar feel like too high a price — that the pull loses its authority.

This moment arrives. Not on a schedule and not at the conclusion of a specific amount of work. But it arrives, for people who do the genuine work, as the lived experience of a pull that used to feel irresistible becoming resistible. Not effortless — resistible. The effort is still present. The pull is still felt. The difference is that the outcome of the encounter with the pull is no longer predetermined.

The unfamiliar peace has to become genuinely compelling for this to happen. Not intellectually preferable — genuinely, experientially, in the body, more attractive than the familiar pain. This requires enough direct experience of the unfamiliar peace that it has accumulated the kind of felt reality that the familiar pain has always had. Which requires staying in it long enough for the nervous system to file it under known. Which requires, for most people, more time in the unfamiliar peace than they initially want to give it, because the initial experience of calm continues to feel like a waiting room rather than a destination.

Stay in the peace long enough to let it become familiar. That is where the cycle breaks — not in understanding but in accumulated experience of something genuinely better.

CHAPTER 17

The Comfort You Found in the Wrong Places

What You Were Actually Looking For in the Things That Hurt You

Reflection 81

The drinking, the relationship that was wrong from the start, the work that consumed you entirely, the distraction that never quite distracted — you were not weak for finding them. You were looking for relief from something that had no other exit.

Every coping mechanism tells a story about the pain it was managing. The specificity of what someone reaches for in their most difficult moments is not random. It corresponds to the precise quality of the relief being sought — the specific feature of the experience that temporarily addresses the most acute dimension of what is being survived.

The alcohol that quieted the hypervigilance — the specific relief of a nervous system that never quite comes down from threat-activation finding the first genuine respite in a substance that chemically overrides the alarm. The relationship that was wrong from the start but felt immediately familiar — the specific recognition of the nervous system encountering the emotional signature it knows how to navigate, however costly that navigation has been. The work that consumed everything — the specific relief of a mind that cannot stop running its pain on repeat finally finding a legitimate reason for total absorption that leaves no attention available for what is actually hurting.

None of these choices were made from strength. They were made from pain. And pain operating without adequate resources and without adequate support makes the best choice available from the options on offer. The options were limited. The pain was real. The choice that provided the most immediate relief was the rational choice in that context.

This is not a defense of the choice's long-term consequences. Some of the consequences were significant and deserve honest acknowledgment. It is a correction of the narrative of weakness — the story that the reaching toward the wrong thing reveals something fundamentally flawed about the person who reached. The person was in pain. The wrong thing offered relief. The reaching made sense.

What also needs to happen is the addressing of the pain that made the wrong thing necessary.

Reflection 82

What you found comfort in was never the problem. The problem was the pain that made you need it.

This distinction matters enormously for what the healing actually requires. If the coping mechanism is the problem, the solution is the elimination of the coping mechanism — the white-knuckled removal of the thing that was providing relief, replaced by nothing or by an affirmation of the superiority of better choices. This approach produces the specific suffering of someone in pain who has had their pain management removed without having their pain addressed.

If the pain is the problem, the solution is the healing of the pain — and the healing of the pain tends to produce, without coercion, the gradual disinterest in the coping mechanism that the pain made necessary. Not in every case and not without additional work in cases where the coping mechanism has developed its own neurological dependency. But as a general orientation, the addressing of the source produces changes in the behavior that the addressing of the behavior alone consistently fails to produce.

The addiction treatment literature is increasingly aligned with this understanding. Gabor Maté's work on addiction as a response to pain rather than a character defect — supported by extensive clinical evidence and developmental research — reframes the question from why the addiction to what pain made the addiction necessary, and consistently finds that the question directed at the source produces better outcomes than the question directed at the behavior.

What was the pain? Specifically and honestly — what was the experience that the coping mechanism was managing? That is the thing that needs tending. When it is tended, the behavior it produced tends to resolve alongside it.

Reflection 83

Judgment of your own coping mechanisms is not healing. Understanding what they were protecting you from is.

The self-judgment is seductive because it provides the specific psychological satisfaction of at least doing something — of not being passive in the face of behavior you want to change. The judgment has energy. It produces the sensation of moral engagement with the problem. It positions you as the person who takes the coping mechanism seriously rather than excusing it.

What it does not do is produce change. The research on shame and behavior is clear on this point — shame reliably produces the motivation to hide, not the motivation to change. The judgment of the coping mechanism activates the shame response, which activates the self-protective impulse, which typically produces either the defensive explanation of the behavior or the doubling-down into it, because the behavior is simultaneously being condemned and providing relief from the condemnation.

Understanding what the coping mechanism was protecting you from requires a different relationship to it — the curious, non-judgmental inquiry of someone who is genuinely trying to understand a behavior rather than convict themselves of it. What did this provide? When did I first reach for it? What was happening in my life at the time that made this response logical? What specific feature of the experience — the numbing, the distraction, the familiar pattern, the total absorption — addressed the most acute dimension of what I was surviving?

The understanding is not permission for the behavior to continue indefinitely. It is the information that makes the behavior comprehensible — which is the prerequisite for addressing it at the level where it was generated rather than at the surface level where the judgment operates and consistently fails.

Reflection 84

You cannot shame yourself into better choices. You can only understand yourself into them.

The self-improvement culture has a complicated and often counterproductive relationship with shame. The specific use of shame as a motivational tool — the before picture, the rock bottom, the confrontation with how bad things have gotten as the mechanism for generating the momentum to change — is predicated on the belief that feeling sufficiently terrible about the current state produces the drive to move toward a different one.

Sometimes it does, in the short term. Shame can produce explosive initial movement. The problem is sustainability. The movement generated by shame requires the continuous feeding of shame to maintain its momentum, which means the person working from shame as their primary motivational fuel is required to sustain a relationship with their own inadequacy as the engine of their progress. And a person in sustained relationship with their own inadequacy is not building the internal foundation that actually supports lasting change. They are building the specific fragility of someone whose motivation evaporates the moment the shame is interrupted by self-compassion.

Understanding produces different movement. It is slower to initiate — understanding requires the patience of genuine inquiry rather than the explosive energy of self-condemnation. But the movement it generates has a different quality. It comes from genuine comprehension of the problem rather than from the aversion to self-judgment. It sustains itself differently because it is not dependent on maintaining a particular relationship with your own inadequacy.

The change you make from genuine understanding of what drove the behavior is a change that can hold through the moments of difficulty, the setbacks, the occasions when the old behavior resurfaces, because the understanding can extend to those moments too — can hold the setback with the same curiosity it brought to the original pattern rather than condemning the setback as evidence that the change was impossible.

Reflection 85

When the wound is addressed, the thing you used to manage it loses its grip. Not always immediately. But the grip loosens. This is how it works.

This is the thing most people do not believe until they experience it, because from inside the grip the loosening feels theoretical — a promise about a future state that is difficult to imagine from the current position. The grip is the entire felt reality. The idea that it loosens is cognitive at best, wishful at worst.

And then it begins to loosen. Not dramatically. The first signs are small — the moment the usual pull toward the coping mechanism arrives and is slightly less insistent than it was last month. The day the craving for the familiar numbing is present but smaller than the craving for the genuine thing it was replacing. The week where the pattern does not activate despite the presence of the usual trigger, which is noticed only in retrospect, which is itself evidence of how thoroughly the loosening has been occurring below the level of conscious tracking.

The loosening happens because the coping mechanism's job is diminishing. When the pain that required the management is being genuinely tended — when the grief is being felt, the anger is being acknowledged, the wound is being entered with adequate support and genuine willingness — the urgency that drove the reaching-for-relief lessens alongside it. Not completely and not immediately and not without the specific work of also addressing whatever neurological dependency the coping mechanism itself has produced. But the root diminishes, and the root's diminishment changes what grows from it.

The grip loosens. This is not wishful thinking. It is the documented pattern of people who do the actual work of addressing the wound rather than the behavior the wound produced.

Tend the wound. Watch what happens to everything that grew from it.

CHAPTER 18

Mistaking Intensity for Love

When Chemistry Was Actually Trauma and Drama Felt Like Connection

Reflection 86

Not everything that felt like electricity was love. Some of it was your nervous system recognizing a familiar pattern of danger and calling it home.

The electricity is real. The neurochemical experience of it — the dopamine spike, the norepinephrine activation, the specific heightened alertness of a nervous system that has encountered something it is wired to pay close attention to — is a genuine physiological event. The feeling is not manufactured or imaginary. It is happening.

What is not reliably true is what the feeling is indicating. The nervous system produces the electricity in response to two very different categories of encounter: genuine connection — the rare experience of meeting someone whose presence activates the social engagement system in the specific way that genuine safety and genuine affinity produce — and familiar danger — the recognition of a pattern that matches the template the nervous system learned to be most alert around.

Both produce electricity. From the inside, they are often indistinguishable. The same heightened awareness. The same sense of this person being somehow more present, more real, more significant than other people. The same quality of being immediately pulled toward rather than having to work toward interest.

The difference is in what follows. Genuine connection deepens into something that feels increasingly safe as it becomes increasingly known. The electricity transforms into warmth, into genuine ease, into the specific quality of being thoroughly known and thoroughly accepted that intimacy is actually designed to produce.

The familiar-danger recognition produces something different. It produces the specific volatility of a dynamic organized around insecurity — the highs and lows, the intensity that looks like passion from the outside and feels like anxiety from the inside, the specific exhaustion of a person whose nervous system has been in threat-response mode for the duration of the relationship while calling the activation love.

Feel the electricity. Then wait to see what it becomes.

Reflection 87

The calm relationship felt boring because calm was unfamiliar. The chaos felt like passion because chaos is what love felt like where you first learned it.

The first template for intimate love is installed before the capacity for critical evaluation of that template. Whatever quality the earliest love relationships had — whatever emotional texture, whatever consistency or inconsistency, whatever the specific felt experience of being in close relationship with the first people who loved you — that quality became the operating definition of what love feels like.

If the first love was calm and consistent and warm and reliable, calm and consistent and warm and reliable feel like love. The nervous system recognizes them as the emotional signature of the original template and responds with the specific ease of a system that has encountered familiar and safe simultaneously.

If the first love was chaotic and conditional and intermittent and activating — if love arrived alongside anxiety, if warmth and withdrawal alternated without predictable logic, if connection required performance and vigilance and the constant management of someone else's emotional state — then that complex of experiences is the template. And what looks like passion in a chaotic adult relationship is the nervous system recognizing the template and calling it home.

The calm partner does not produce the activation because the calm partner does not match the template. The calm, the reliability, the genuine steadiness feel like something is missing — because in the template, something was always in danger of being withdrawn, and the absence of that threat does not register as safety. It registers as flatness.

The boredom is not information about the relationship. It is information about the template. And the template can be updated — through the specific, extended, patient experience of staying in the calm relationship long enough for the nervous system to file calm under love.

Reflection 88

When you heal what taught you that love was supposed to hurt, the relationships that are actually good for you will start to feel like what they are — not boring, but safe. And safe, it turns out, is what you were looking for the whole time.

The recalibration is not instantaneous. The person who has spent years oriented toward the activating, the familiar-danger, the emotionally intense does not simply decide to find the calm relationship compelling and find it so. The recalibration happens through the work — through the addressing of the original wound that installed the dangerous-feels-like-love template, through the accumulated experience of choosing the calm relationship in spite of the initial absence of the activation it was expected to produce, through the gradual discovery that what felt like flatness at the beginning is revealing itself, over time and over the specific deepening that genuine consistency produces, as something with a texture the chaos never provided.

The chaos never actually provided what was being sought in it. The chaos provided activation — the specific feeling of aliveness that a nervous system in threat-response generates, which is intense and consuming and mistakable for passion, but which is not connection. It is threat-response. And threat-response, sustained over the duration of a relationship, produces not intimacy but the specific exhaustion of a person who has been in flight-or-fight mode while believing they were in love.

The calm relationship that reveals itself as genuinely good — as the relationship where your full self is welcome, where repair happens without destruction, where consistency produces depth rather than the boredom the template predicted — that relationship feels, over time, like nothing the chaos could touch.

Not boring. Safe. Deeply, genuinely, irreversibly safe.

And safe — the thing the nervous system has been seeking through every dangerous thing it ever called home — is the thing you were looking for the whole time.

***

"She had mistaken electricity for connection for so long that when genuine warmth finally arrived, she almost left because it did not hurt enough to feel real. She stayed just long enough to discover that real had never required hurting at all."

PART SIX: BECOMING SOMEONE WHO DOES NOT BETRAY HERSELF

Building the Internal Foundation That Makes Self-Loyalty Possible

CHAPTER 19

Learning to Trust Yourself Again

Rebuilding the Relationship With Your Own Instincts After Years of Ignoring Them

Reflection 89

Every time you overrode your instinct and the instinct was right, you made a withdrawal from your self-trust account. The account is low. You can rebuild it.

The account does not close. That is the first thing worth knowing. However depleted it has become — however many years of accumulated overrides have reduced the balance to something that barely registers — the account remains open and it responds to deposits the same way it always did. One honest, instinct-honored decision at a time.

Think about the withdrawals. Not to punish yourself for making them — they were made for reasons that made sense in the context that produced them. But to understand the scale of what has been withdrawn, because the scale of the depletion explains the current balance without making it permanent.

Every time the gut said something is wrong here and the mind found six reasonable explanations for why the gut was probably overreacting — withdrawal. Every time the body tensed in the presence of a specific person and the decision was made to override the tension because the tension seemed disproportionate or unkind or not sufficiently evidenced — withdrawal. Every time the clear perception arrived ahead of the justification and was talked out of itself before it had time to become actionable — withdrawal.

Years of this produces a specific relationship with your own knowing. Not the absence of the knowing — the instinct does not stop generating accurate information because it has been repeatedly ignored. But the absence of trust in the knowing. The reflex of doubt that arrives alongside the instinct, the immediate question of whether this one is real or whether this is the anxiety, the specific paralysis of someone who can feel the signal but can no longer reliably determine whether the signal warrants response.

The account rebuilds through deposits. Small ones first. The next instinct honored, even in a low-stakes moment. Then the next. The balance grows slowly and the trust that grows with it is real — not assumed, not borrowed from someone else's assessment of your judgment, but earned through the accumulated evidence of your own reliable perception.

Reflection 90

Your instincts were not wrong. They were inconvenient. There is a significant difference.

The environments that trained you to distrust your instincts had a specific investment in that distrust. Your accurate perception of what was happening was inconvenient to the people whose behavior your perception was accurately pointing at. Your clear-eyed reading of the dynamic was a problem for the dynamic's continuation. Your instinct that something was wrong was a direct threat to the story that everything was fine.

So the instinct was relabeled. Not wrong in the sense of being inaccurate — the people doing the relabeling often knew, at some level, that the instinct was accurate. Wrong in the sense of being inappropriate. Too sensitive. Too reactive. Not fair to the person the perception was directed at. Evidence of your anxiety rather than their behavior. Evidence of your tendency to make things difficult rather than their behavior that warranted the response you were having.

The relabeling worked. Not permanently, but sufficiently — long enough and consistently enough that you began applying it yourself. You began doing the work of doubting your own perception before anyone else had to do it for you. You became expert at the preemptive override — the self-administered correction that kept the inconvenient perception from becoming visible, kept the dynamic intact, kept the peace at the price of your own accurate knowing.

The instinct was not wrong. It was pointing at things that were real and that certain people needed you to be unable to see clearly. The doubt was installed in service of their comfort, not your accuracy. Recovering the trust in your instincts is recovering the accuracy that was always there — not a new capacity, but the one you were talked out of.

Reflection 91

Start with the small things. Trust yourself about what you want for dinner, which friend to call, when you need to leave. The trust rebuilds from the small before it is available for the large.

The restoration of self-trust has to be graduated because the nervous system learns through accumulated evidence, and evidence accumulates one instance at a time. Asking a self-trust account depleted by years of override to immediately handle the large, consequential decisions — the relationship, the career, the significant life choice — is asking depleted infrastructure to carry a load it has not yet been rebuilt to support.

Start where the stakes are low and the evidence is fast. The preference for dinner is a clean, immediate, low-consequence trust-exercise — you identify what you want, you choose it, you discover whether the choice served you, the feedback loop closes quickly and clearly. The decision about which friend to call when something difficult is happening — trusting the name that comes first rather than running it through the analysis of who should be called. The moment in a social situation when the body says it is time to leave — acting on that signal rather than overriding it for the sake of not disrupting the evening.

Each of these small acts of honored instinct adds to the account. Each one produces the specific, small, cumulative evidence that your perception is reliable — that when you identify what you want, the choosing of it generally serves you. That when your body signals a preference or a limit, respecting the signal produces better outcomes than overriding it.

The large decisions do not wait forever. But they become available more reliably, with less paralysis, when they arrive at a self-trust account that has been rebuilt through the patient accumulation of small deposits. The foundation matters. Build it from the small things and the large ones become less precarious.

Reflection 92

The voice you have been overriding is not the enemy. It is the most honest thing about you. It deserves a hearing.

The internal voice that generates clear knowing before the reasoning catches up — the one that said something is wrong and was talked out of it, the one that said this is not right for me and was overridden by the list of reasons it should be right, the one that said leave and was silenced by the accumulated weight of everything that staying required — that voice has been one of the most reliable and most consistently ignored sources of information available to you.

It is not anxiety. Anxiety generates catastrophic projections about imagined futures. The instinct-voice is specific, present-tense, and attached to direct perception rather than to narrative elaboration. It does not say this will end badly in some unspecified future. It says something is off right now, in this specific interaction, about this specific thing. The specificity is the tell. Anxiety is general. Instinct is precise.

It is not paranoia. Paranoia is suspicious of everything and attached to no particular evidence. The instinct-voice arises in response to specific inputs — specific behaviors, specific tones, specific moments where the presented version of events does not match the felt version of events — and it subsides when those inputs are no longer present. It tracks reality rather than manufacturing threat in the absence of it.

The voice you have been overriding has been accurate more than you have been willing to acknowledge. Not perfectly accurate — no perceptual system is. But accurate enough, consistently enough, that the pattern of its accuracy deserves your attention.

Give it a hearing. Not automatic compliance — the voice is one input, not the only input. But genuine consideration, without the immediate deployment of the doubt-mechanism that has been silencing it. Let it speak. Then assess what it is saying with the honest curiosity of someone who has finally decided that what they perceive is worth taking seriously.

Reflection 93

You will not trust yourself perfectly immediately. You will trust yourself imperfectly and keep going. The imperfect practice is the whole thing.

The expectation of perfect self-trust before the practicing begins is the same structure as every other version of waiting to be ready before starting. It places the resource downstream of the practice that builds it, which means it remains permanently unavailable until the practice is undertaken anyway, imperfectly, without the resource fully in place.

You will honor an instinct and discover it was off. Not often — the instinct is more reliable than the doubt mechanism has allowed you to believe — but sometimes, because no perceptual system is infallible and because rebuilding trust requires the same room for error that any learning process requires. The occasional error is not evidence that the trust was misplaced. It is evidence that you are a person with imperfect perception, which is the condition of all people, and that imperfect perception trusted and calibrated over time produces better outcomes than accurate perception routinely suppressed.

You will override the instinct occasionally even as you are working to trust it. The old habits have deep grooves. The override reflex will activate before you have had time to catch it, especially in high-stakes or emotionally loaded situations where the nervous system defaults to its most practiced response. The goal is not zero overrides. The goal is a decreasing ratio — more instances of honored instinct and fewer of reflexive suppression, moved toward gradually and imperfectly and with the specific patience of someone building something that takes time.

The imperfect practice is the whole thing. Not the perfected version that you might get to eventually. The current imperfect practice, undertaken consistently, is the mechanism of the change you are working toward.

CHAPTER 20

The Identity That Exists Beyond the Suffering

Who You Are When the Pain Is No Longer the Defining Feature

Reflection 94

You have been so long in the wound that you may have confused it with your identity. You are not your history. You are what you do with it.

Identity and history are not the same thing. History is the record of what occurred — the events, the relationships, the experiences that shaped the person who is here now. Identity is what is happening in the person who is here now — the values, the capacities, the specific quality of engagement with the world that constitutes the ongoing, living, continuously developing self.

The wound is history. The identity organized around the wound is the confusion — the collapsing of what happened into who you are, which produces the specific stuckness of a person who cannot imagine herself outside the context of her damage because she has been inside it long enough that the context has become the definition.

Viktor Frankl survived Auschwitz. He wrote, from direct experience of the most extreme available conditions, that the last of human freedoms is the ability to choose one's attitude toward any given set of circumstances. He was not denying the reality of what happened or the profound shaping it produced. He was insisting on the space between what happens and who is responding to it — the space where identity lives, separate from history, making of the history something that history alone cannot determine.

What happened to you is real. What it produced in you is real. Neither of these facts is the final word on who you are, because who you are is not a fixed conclusion derived from the available evidence of your history. It is an ongoing project — shaped by history, not owned by it. Available for development, for revision, for the specific becoming that happens when the wound is no longer required to be the center of everything.

The identity beyond the suffering is not yet fully known. That is not a problem. It is the invitation.

Reflection 95

The woman on the other side of this does not have a perfect life. She has a genuine one — built from honesty rather than performance, from choice rather than survival.

The fantasy of what the healed life looks like is usually too clean. The unburdened ease, the relationships that work without friction, the absence of difficulty, the specific luminosity of a person who has gotten through something and arrived somewhere good and settled. This fantasy is understandable — when you are in significant pain, the imagination of its absence tends toward the absolute. No more of this, and everything that follows is better.

The reality of the healed life is less dramatic and more sustaining than the fantasy. Not the absence of difficulty — difficulty is a permanent feature of human existence and the healing does not exempt you from it. Not the absence of pain — pain is the accurate signal of things that matter and the healing does not anesthetize it. Not the arrival at some final version of yourself that no longer requires tending.

What the healed life actually looks like is the ordinary life lived with genuine presence rather than managed from behind performance. The difficult conversation had rather than swallowed. The limit held rather than dissolved under pressure. The relationship that can hold the full texture of two actual people because neither person is required to manage the other's capacity for reality. The morning that begins without the specific weight of a life organized around pain — which does not feel dramatic, which feels like ordinary Tuesday, which is exactly what it is.

That ordinary Tuesday — lived genuinely, from choice, from honesty, from the specific groundedness of a self who knows herself and trusts herself and no longer requires the suffering to feel real — is worth more than the dramatic fantasy of the healed life. It is what the healed life actually is. And it is available.

Reflection 96

You will not know who you are without the suffering until you have lived without it long enough to find out. The finding out is the most interesting part.

Most people approach this discovery with anxiety. The not-knowing feels threatening — the loss of the familiar identity without the immediate availability of the replacement produces the specific disorientation of someone between selves. Not yet the old one, which is dissolving. Not yet the new one, which has not fully formed. Standing in the gap with less certainty about who is standing there than has been available in a long time.

The anxiety is understandable. The gap is real. And the anxiety, while present, does not have to determine the relationship you have to the gap. The gap is also the space where discovery is possible — where the qualities that were suppressed by the wound's requirements begin to surface, where the preferences that were managed into invisibility begin to become legible, where the person who exists without the suffering as her defining context begins to reveal herself in the specific, surprising, genuinely interesting detail of an actual individual rather than an organized-around-damage prototype.

Some of what you discover will be immediately recognizable — qualities you knew were there but that had not had adequate room to develop inside the wound-organized life. Some will be genuinely surprising — capacities and preferences and ways of engaging with the world that you had no idea were present because the wound was occupying the space they would otherwise have inhabited.

The finding out is the most interesting part. Not the part before it — the suffering has rarely been described as interesting. Not the part after it — the settled, integrated life has its own richness but lacks the specific aliveness of genuine discovery. The finding out itself — the emergence of the self that has been waiting — is the part that makes the whole difficult process worth exactly what it cost.

Reflection 97

Some of what you discover about yourself on the other side will surprise you. Some of it you already knew. All of it has been waiting.

The things you already knew will arrive first, usually. The preferences that were suppressed rather than absent. The capacities that were present but underexpressed. The qualities — the humor, the directness, the specific ways of engaging with the world that felt too much or too risky to fully inhabit inside the wound-organized life — that were always there and begin to surface with increasing confidence as the pressure that kept them managed is lifted.

These feel like coming home to rooms you had forgotten were part of the house. The recognition is immediate. The relief is specific. The specific quality of these qualities being finally, fully expressed — without the management, without the calculation of whether it is safe to bring them into the current context — feels less like discovery and more like return.

The surprising things arrive later, and they are more interesting. The creative capacity that had no room. The appetite for risk or adventure or genuine engagement with the world that the wound's demands had crowded out entirely. The quality of presence that becomes available when the threat-assessment system is no longer required to be continuously active. The specific, deeply personal ways that the person who is not organized around pain engages with the experiences, the relationships, the ordinary details of daily life.

These are not qualities you can predict from inside the wound because the wound was occupying the space they require. They only become visible when the space is cleared. They are real — not wishes, not projections, but the actual, present, genuinely yours dimensions of a self that was always more complex and more interesting than the wound allowed her to be.

They have been waiting. The waiting is ending.

Reflection 98

You are not rebuilding a self. You are uncovering one. She was always there under everything that covered her.

The rebuilding metaphor suggests that what the wound did was destroy the self — that what remains in the aftermath is rubble, and the work is construction from the ground up, which is an enormous and daunting project that can feel impossible when the available resources are already depleted by the work of survival.

The uncovering metaphor is more accurate and considerably less daunting. What the wound did was not destroy the self. It covered her. It accumulated, over years of adaptive response to difficult conditions, layers of performance and management and protective mechanism that served a genuine purpose and that now obscure the self rather than constituting her.

She did not disappear under the covering. She waited. The curiosity that was managed into appropriate modesty. The ambition that was judged into modesty of a different kind. The voice that was trained into silence. The preferences that were overridden into invisibility. The specific, irreplaceable, entirely individual self who would have developed more freely in different conditions — she is still there, under the layers, intact in the ways that matter most.

The work is not construction. It is the careful, patient, sometimes arduous removal of what covered her. Each layer of performed identity released. Each protective mechanism examined and, where it no longer serves, set aside. Each self-betrayal corrected in the moment of noticing rather than the moment after.

As the covering is removed, she becomes more visible. More available. More present in the daily experience of a life that is beginning to fit her rather than containing her.

She was always there. Now she gets to be seen.

CHAPTER 21

Choosing Yourself in Real Time

What Self-Loyalty Looks Like as a Daily Practice, Not a One-Time Decision

Reflection 99

Loyalty to yourself is not a dramatic declaration. It is Thursday afternoon when everything is pulling at you and you choose the thing that actually serves you anyway.

The dramatic declaration has its place. The moment of genuine commitment — the decision, made with clarity and intention, to stop organizing your life around your own suffering — is real and it matters and it deserves to be acknowledged as the beginning of something significant.

And then Thursday arrives. With its competing demands and its ordinary friction and its specific accumulation of the small moments where the old patterns reassert themselves with the comfortable efficiency of long practice. Thursday does not care about the dramatic declaration. Thursday presents the usual cast of situations that have historically produced the self-betraying response, and it waits to see what happens.

Thursday is where the loyalty is built or not built. In the small choice made correctly when nobody is watching and nothing particularly significant is at stake and the old response would be so much easier than the new one and the new one requires the specific effort of doing something against the grain of years of conditioning.

The rest taken on Thursday afternoon when the guilt says there is more to do. The email not sent on Thursday evening when the boundary is challenged and the familiar response would be to smooth it over. The conversation had on Thursday over dinner when the thing needed to be said and the history of swallowing it was pressing strongly and it got said anyway.

These Thursdays accumulate into a life. Not the dramatic life of the single transformative decision. The actual life — built from the ordinary moments where the loyalty is either practiced or deferred, and where the practice, sustained across ordinary Thursday after ordinary Thursday, becomes who you are.

Reflection 100

It is the conversation you have instead of the one you swallow. The rest you take instead of the productivity you perform. The no that holds instead of the yes that costs you.

Self-loyalty in practice is almost always smaller than the idea of it suggests. The grand narratives around self-care and self-prioritization tend to involve sweeping changes, complete reinventions, dramatic departures from the previous life. These things happen sometimes. More often, what changes is the texture of the ordinary — the specific quality of the small daily decisions that, accumulated across a life, constitute what the life actually was.

The conversation you have instead of swallowing is rarely the one you have been rehearsing for months. It is more often the smaller truth, stated in the ordinary moment — the correction offered instead of the agreement performed, the need expressed instead of denied, the honest response given instead of the managed one. Small. Real. Repeated.

The rest taken instead of productivity performed does not arrive as a sweeping restructuring of your relationship with work and rest. It arrives as the Tuesday afternoon when you close the computer thirty minutes earlier than the guilt says is acceptable, and you do not spend the thirty minutes justifying the decision to yourself. Small. Real. Repeated.

The no that holds instead of the yes that costs is not the grand limit-setting that goes into the self-help books. It is the ordinary no that arrives in response to an ordinary ask and that stays no through the first moment of pushback rather than softening immediately into a qualified yes. Small. Real. Repeated.

These are the acts. Not impressive from the outside. Irreplaceable from the inside. The life is built from them.

Reflection 101

Some days the most loyal thing you can do for yourself is refuse to add to your own suffering by being unkind to yourself about how the healing is going.

The secondary suffering — the suffering generated by the judgment of the primary suffering — is optional. The primary suffering is what happened and what it produced and what it continues to produce as the healing moves through it. That suffering has genuine causes and genuine weight and deserves genuine acknowledgment and genuine tending.

The judgment of the primary suffering is the addition on top — the self-criticism about being too slow, the comparison to other people's timelines, the verdict that not being further along by now is evidence of inadequacy, the specific unkindness of a person who is already in pain and is also holding herself to a standard that the pain itself makes impossible to meet.

On the days when the healing feels stuck, when the old patterns have reasserted themselves, when the progress that seemed solid has become temporarily less visible — the most genuinely self-loyal available choice is often not a new strategy or a more committed effort or a harder push through the current difficulty. It is the cessation of the unkindness. The simple withdrawal of the judgment that you are failing at something you are in the middle of doing.

You are not failing. You are in it. The difference between those two assessments is the difference between unnecessary additional suffering and the specific, hard-earned peace of someone who is doing difficult work and has decided to be decent to themselves while doing it.

Decency toward yourself in the middle of the difficulty is not the lowering of standards. It is the basic condition under which genuine healing can actually proceed.

Reflection 102

You will relapse into the old patterns. That is not the end of the work. That is the work — noticing, returning, choosing again.

The relapse is built into the structure of the change, not evidence against it. Neural patterns developed over years of consistent activation do not disappear after months of practicing the alternative. They become less dominant, less automatic, less likely to determine the outcome when the trigger arrives — and in the meantime, they remain accessible, particularly under conditions of high stress, high fatigue, or the specific emotional activation that the original wound is most sensitive to.

The relapse will feel like failure. Every time. Regardless of how clearly you understand the mechanism, regardless of how many times you have been here before and found your way back, the specific quality of being back in the old pattern after the work of getting out of it carries the emotional weight of defeat.

That weight is not accurate. The relapse is data — specific information about the conditions under which the old pattern is still strong enough to override the new one, about what the current work most needs to address, about where the new pattern requires additional support. It is not a verdict on the work's ultimate success. It is a checkpoint in a process that is not linear and that never promised to be.

The thing that actually ends the pattern is not the first departure from it. It is the thousandth return after the relapse. The noticing — I am here again — without the catastrophizing. The returning — this is what I am working toward — without the self-condemnation for having departed. The choosing again — the different choice made from exactly this position of having just been in the old place — which is the most powerful version of the choice available, because it is made with full knowledge of the cost and full choice anyway.

Notice. Return. Choose again. That is the whole practice.

Reflection 103

The practice of self-loyalty is the practice of treating yourself as someone whose experience matters, whose needs are real, and whose suffering is not a life sentence.

Strip away the language around self-care and boundaries and healing, and what the practice of self-loyalty actually requires is something simpler and more radical than any of the specific techniques: the daily, practiced, continuously renewed decision to include yourself in the category of people who matter.

Not above everyone else. Not at the expense of genuine care for the people in your life. Inside the same category — the category of beings whose experience is real and whose needs deserve genuine consideration and whose suffering is worth addressing rather than being organized around as though it were simply the permanent condition of their existence.

You have been excluding yourself from that category. Not in a single decision but in the accumulated pattern of ten thousand small ones — every time your experience was the variable that got cut when the budget ran tight, every time your need was the one that went unaddressed when the logistics of addressing everyone else's were complete, every time your suffering was the one that did not get tended because you were busy tending everyone else's.

The practice of including yourself is the correction of that pattern. One ordinary moment at a time. The moment when you notice your experience and let it be real before moving to address everyone else's. The moment when you identify a need and bring it the same quality of genuine response you would bring to someone else's. The moment when you recognize the suffering and turn toward it rather than past it.

That practice, sustained, becomes character. And character, sustained, becomes a life.

CHAPTER 22

The Life That Becomes Available When You Stop Betraying Yourself

What Waits on the Other Side of Self-Loyalty

Reflection 104

The life available on the other side of self-betrayal is not a fantasy. It is ordinary and real and genuinely yours — built from choices made in your own interest for the first time.

The ordinariness is the part nobody prepares you for. The life that becomes available when the self-betrayal ends does not arrive with cinematic quality. It does not produce the specific luminosity of the transformation narrative or the dramatic contrast of the before-and-after. It arrives quietly, incrementally, in the accumulation of ordinary days that have a different quality than the ordinary days that preceded them.

The difference is in the texture. The morning that begins without the specific weight of a life organized around what hurts you. Not a perfect morning — mornings are still mornings, with their ordinary friction and their ordinary demands. But a morning where the weight is different. Where the energy available for the day is not already depleted by the maintenance of the suffering. Where the body is not already in threat-response before the day has properly begun.

The relationships that carry a different quality — not because the people have changed, but because the terms of your participation in them have. The conversation that is honest rather than managed. The limit that holds rather than dissolves. The genuine presence of a person who is actually in the relationship rather than performing inside it.

The work that has a different relationship to your worth — where the doing of it is not required to prove something or compensate for something or distract from something, but is simply the expression of genuine capacity applied to something that matters.

This is the life. Ordinary. Real. Genuinely yours. It was available all along, on the other side of the betrayal of yourself that was preventing you from inhabiting it.

Reflection 105

You will not recognize yourself immediately. Give it time. The woman who does not betray herself is quieter than you expected. Less anxious. More present. More here.

The version of yourself that you will become through this work is not the version the fantasy produced. The fantasy version tends toward a kind of confident luminosity — the woman who has done the work and arrived somewhere and knows it and carries that knowing with a visible assurance that reads as healed. The actual version is quieter. Less dramatic. More genuinely present in the specific moment she is actually in rather than managing three moments simultaneously.

The quietness surprises people. When the threat-assessment system is no longer running continuously — when the nervous system is no longer scanning for danger in every interaction, no longer preparing for the withdrawal of love or the approach of harm — the specific volume of the internal environment decreases. Not the richness. The anxiety-noise. The specific hum of a system that has been in low-level activation for so long that the activation had become indistinguishable from consciousness itself.

In its absence, something more subtle is available. The actual texture of the present moment, without the overlay of threat-response and management. The specific quality of genuine presence with another person, without the simultaneous processing of what they might need and what might need to be managed and whether the current interaction is safe. The experience of your own thoughts and perceptions without the immediate editorial layer that assessed their acceptability before allowing them to be real.

The woman who does not betray herself is more here than the woman who did. Less spectacular from the outside, perhaps. More genuinely alive from the inside, without question. Give it time to become familiar. The quiet is not emptiness. It is what genuine presence actually feels like.

Reflection 106

The relationships that find you on the other side of this work will be different — not because the world changed but because you stopped accepting what you used to accept as the price of admission.

The world does not change. The people in it remain as they were — with their own wounds, their own patterns, their own specific capacity for genuine connection and their own specific limitations. What changes is the filter through which you engage with them — the standard against which what is offered is assessed, the specific quality of presence you bring that makes certain kinds of relationship possible and others impossible to sustain.

The relationships organized around your self-betrayal — the ones that required your smallness, your silence, your unlimited availability, your willingness to receive less than you were giving — those relationships change when you change. Some of them shift and become something more genuinely mutual, because the people in them have more capacity than the old dynamic revealed and your change creates the conditions for their genuine response. Some of them dissolve, because the dynamic was the entire content and the dynamic is no longer available.

The new relationships — the ones that find the changed version of you rather than the betraying version — have a different quality from the beginning. Not perfect. Not without the ordinary friction of two actual people learning each other. But organized around something real rather than around your performance of someone who requires nothing.

The price of admission to these relationships is your presence, not your disappearance. Your honesty, not your management. Your actual self, offered genuinely rather than curated for palatability.

That price is the one you can afford. It is, in fact, the only one you can afford indefinitely.

Reflection 107

What you could not imagine from inside the suffering — that peace could be real, that calm could feel like home, that you could exist without the weight — becomes ordinary. That ordinariness is not a disappointment. It is the whole point.

From inside significant, sustained suffering, peace is genuinely difficult to imagine as a felt experience. You can describe it. You can understand it conceptually. But the felt reality of it — what it actually feels like in the body to be a person who is not organized around her own pain — is not available as imagination from inside the experience that makes it its opposite.

This is why so many people pursue healing without being entirely sure what they are moving toward. They know the direction — away from this — without being able to fully imagine the destination. They are trusting that something better exists on the other side of the work without the specific experiential evidence of what better actually feels like.

The trust is warranted. What becomes available on the other side is not the dramatic transformation the suffering-imagination produced as its fantasy. It is more ordinary than that, and the ordinariness is not the compromise version of what was hoped for. It is what genuine peace actually is.

Peace is the Tuesday that passes without the specific weight. The night that ends without the specific anxiety. The ordinary interaction that occurs without the specific threat-assessment overlay. The experience of being alive in your own life without the particular heaviness of a life organized around what hurts you.

The ordinariness is the point. Not because ordinary is small. Because ordinary, lived from genuine groundedness rather than performed from exhausted maintenance, is the most sustaining quality of existence available. The dramatic life is exhausting. The genuine life — ordinary, real, unperformed — is what you were looking for all along.

Reflection 108

You stop suffering loyally the same way you started — one small, honest, courageous choice at a time. Except now the choices are different. And so are you.

The starting was not dramatic either. It accumulated — one small self-abandonment at a time, one quiet override of the instinct, one unmeant yes, one swallowed truth, until the pattern was established and the suffering was home and the loyalty to it was the organizing principle of a life.

The stopping mirrors the starting in its structure and reverses it in its direction. One small honest choice at a time. One instinct honored where it used to be overridden. One truth expressed where it used to be managed into silence. One limit held where it used to dissolve under the first pressure. One need acknowledged where it used to be denied before it had time to become fully conscious.

These are the same small moments the suffering was built from, moving now in the opposite direction. Not dramatically. Not with the fanfare of transformation narratives. With the same quiet accumulation that built the pattern, now applied to its dismantling.

The choices are different now because you are different. Not completely different — the work does not produce a new person unrelated to the previous one. Genuinely different. More honest with yourself than before. More willing to feel what is actually happening than to manage it into the acceptable version. More capable of the pause between trigger and response where the different choice lives. More trusting of the voice that has always known and that is finally being heard.

You stopped suffering loyally the way it happened — gradually, in ordinary moments, through the patient accumulation of small honest choices made differently than they used to be.

The suffering was never going to end in a single dramatic decision. Neither is this.

It is ending now, in this moment, in the next one, in the one after that.

One choice at a time.

CHAPTER 23

No Longer Loyal — The Final Reflections

What It Means to Finally Choose Differently

Reflection 109

The suffering was never who you were. It was what happened to you. And what happens to you and who you are have always been two different things — even when the line between them was impossible to find.

The conflation of suffering and identity is one of the wound's most lasting effects and one of the most important things to be clear about before closing this book. Because the conflation does not end automatically when the healing begins. It has to be consciously, repeatedly, sometimes forcefully undone — the story that what happened is who you are has to be met with the specific and consistent counter-story that it is not.

What happened was real. Profoundly real. Formative in ways that are visible throughout everything this book has addressed — in the patterns, the coping mechanisms, the relational templates, the specific quality of the relationship with your own suffering that has been the book's subject. The shaping was genuine and significant and deserves honest acknowledgment rather than minimization.

And the shaping is not the self. The self is what has been navigating, surviving, adapting, and — through this work — beginning to choose differently in response to the shaping. The self is the agency inside the history, not its product. The self is the one doing the work of this book, which is itself the evidence that the self exists separately from the suffering — because the suffering cannot do the work of ending the loyalty to itself. Only the self can do that.

You exist separately from your history. You always have, even in the periods when the separation was invisible. The suffering happened to you. It did not become you. It is not you now.

You are the one who survived it and is choosing, with the specific courage of someone who knows exactly what the old choice cost, something different.

That choosing is who you are. Not the suffering. The response to it.

Reflection 110

This is not the end of difficulty. It is the end of choosing it on your behalf. The end of organizing your life around what hurts you. The end of the loyalty that was costing you everything and giving you nothing in return. You are no longer loyal to your suffering. You are loyal to yourself now. Finally. Completely. Without apology. That changes everything.

Difficulty does not end. This needs to be said plainly, because the healing process can produce the expectation that its completion delivers exemption — that the work done grants some protection from the ordinary and extraordinary hardships of human existence. It does not. Loss will still arrive. Relationships will still carry friction. Health will still be temporary. Uncertainty will still be the permanent condition of a life being lived forward into an unknown future.

What ends is something specific and enormously significant: the addition of the chosen suffering on top of the unavoidable difficulty. The relationships organized around your pain that required your ongoing diminishment as their operating condition. The patterns that recreated the wound because the wound remained unaddressed. The daily, accumulated self-betrayals that kept the suffering alive and familiar and mistakable for home. The loyalty to your own pain that was consuming the energy, the attention, the genuine presence that your actual life deserved and was not receiving.

That loyalty ends. Not in a single moment of arrival — the work is ongoing, the practice is daily, the returning to yourself after each departure is the permanent requirement of a life genuinely inhabited rather than performed. But the direction has changed. The organizing principle has shifted. The central loyalty is no longer to the suffering.

It is to yourself.

To the specific, imperfect, genuinely yours self who has been under the suffering all along — who survived what tried to define her, who did the work of refusing to let it, who is choosing now, in this moment and the next one and the one after that, the different life that the different loyalty makes possible.

You are no longer loyal to your suffering.

That is not a small thing. That is the whole thing.

Everything that follows from it is the life you were always supposed to be living.

Go live it.

***

"She did not leave her suffering in a single dramatic moment. She left it the same way she had entered it — gradually, in small honest choices, one ordinary day at a time. Until the day she looked back and

realized she had not been there in a while. And for the first time, the absence felt not like loss but like the specific, irreversible relief of someone who has finally, completely, come home to herself."

EPILOGUE

A Letter to the Woman Who Survived Herself and Chose to Stay

You made it through this book. That is not a small thing.

Not because reading is difficult. Because what this book asked of you was not passive. It asked you to sit with things that most people spend enormous energy avoiding — the honest accounting of where the suffering came from and what it cost and how long you kept choosing it and what role you played in the keeping. It asked you to look at yourself clearly, without the protective layer of self-pity that makes the looking easier and without the protective layer of self-blame that makes it feel like you are at least doing something. It asked for something considerably harder than either of those: the honest, compassionate, unflinching witness to your own story.

If you did that — if you moved through these pages with genuine engagement rather than comfortable distance — something has shifted. Not everything. Not permanently, without further work. But something, in the specific way that honest reckoning shifts things before the behavioral change has fully arrived, before the new patterns have replaced the old, before the healing is visible from the outside or even entirely legible from the inside.

The shift is real. Trust it. It is the ground that the rest of the work gets built on.

There is something I want to say to you directly, before this book closes, that the format of reflections did not quite make room for.

You survived yourself. Not just the people who hurt you, not just the circumstances that were difficult, not just the wound that was installed before you were old enough to question it. You survived the version of yourself that was keeping you inside the suffering. The internal critic who turned the anger inward. The self-doubt that overrode the accurate instinct. The guilt that reversed the necessary limit. The story that made the staying feel required. The loyalty to your own pain that functioned, for years, as its own kind of home.

Surviving those things — from the inside, without the drama of an external villain to organize the narrative around — is one of the more demanding versions of surviving that exists. The wound from outside is at least clearly located. The wound administered internally, through the accumulated self-betrayals that this book has been naming, is harder to see and harder to leave precisely because the person causing it and the person experiencing it are the same person, sharing the same body, the same history, the same genuine desire to be okay.

You did not know, for a long time, that you were doing it. Or you knew and could not yet stop. Or you stopped and started again, repeatedly, without the specific internal resources that stopping sustainably requires. All of those are versions of the same story — a person who was in more pain than she had adequate support for, managing the best way available, looking for the exit with insufficient equipment for the finding.

You found better equipment. Possibly in this book, possibly in the therapy or the relationship or the conversation or the moment of quiet honesty that preceded this book and made it land the way it did. Wherever the equipment was built, you built it. Nobody hands that to you. You accumulate it through the specific, effortful, unglamorous work of honest self-examination that most people are too frightened to sustain.

Now I want to say the thing that gets left out of most books on healing, because most books end with the arrival — with the message that the work is done and the life is different and the woman has become who she was always meant to be.

The work is not done.

The work will not be done for as long as you are alive and choosing and human, because living requires choosing and choosing requires the ongoing practice of self-loyalty in the specific ordinary moments that constitute a life. The healing is not an achieved state. It is a practice — the daily, imperfect, continuously renewable practice of treating yourself as someone who deserves to be in your own corner.

Some days that practice will be easy. The new patterns will have sufficient momentum, the self-trust will be sufficiently rebuilt, the quality of your relationships will reflect the changes you have made with enough clarity that the practice feels less like effort and more like simply being who you are now.

Some days it will be hard. The old patterns will reassert themselves with the specific authority of long practice. The guilt will be loud. The instinct will be challenged by someone who benefits from your doubting it. The limit will be tested by someone who preferred the limitless version. The suffering will feel, in specific activated moments, more like home than the peace you have been building.

On those days, come back to this. Not necessarily to these pages — though you are welcome to return to whatever reflection most clearly names what is happening on that particular day. Come back to the essential thing this book has been pointing at:

You are not loyal to the suffering anymore. Even when the suffering is loud and the loyalty is tempting and everything in you that was built inside the wound is pulling toward the familiar painful home.

You are loyal to yourself.

That loyalty does not have to be perfect to be real. It does not have to be without relapse or without the occasional day when the old pattern wins the moment. It has to be the direction — the consistent, renewed, day-by-day orientation toward your own genuine wellbeing that makes the relapse an interruption rather than a conclusion, that makes the hard day one day in a life that is genuinely moving in a different direction.

Keep moving in that direction.

Not because it is easy. Not because you will always be certain it is right. Not because the world will reliably reward you for it or because everyone in your life will respond to your growth with the generous welcome it deserves. Because the alternative — the life organized around your own suffering, the loyalty to what hurts you, the daily self-betrayal that was so thoroughly practiced it stopped registering as betrayal — because that alternative cost you something you cannot afford to keep paying.

It cost you your presence in your own life. Your genuine inhabitation of your own experience. The specific, irreplaceable texture of being a person who is actually here, actually choosing, actually alive in the days she is living rather than managing them from behind the protective layer of a self that learned to produce fine as its primary output regardless of what was actually happening underneath.

You survived yourself. You chose to stay — not in the suffering, but in the work of leaving it. Not in the familiar painful home, but in the unfamiliar, occasionally disorienting, genuinely yours life that becomes available when the loyalty finally turns in the right direction.

That staying is extraordinary. Even when it feels ordinary. Even when it feels like just getting through the week. The choosing, sustained across ordinary weeks, is the most significant thing a person can do.

You are doing it.

Keep going.

With genuine respect for what you survived and deep faith in what you are becoming —

This book

ACKNOWLEDGMENTS & GRATITUDE

Books about suffering are made from the people willing to be honest about theirs.

This book exists because of women who told the truth about what it cost them to stay loyal to their own pain — in therapy rooms and journaling pages and the specific late-night hours when pretending gets too heavy to maintain. Women who sat with me in the middle of their own reckonings and allowed me to witness what that actually looks like — not the polished retrospective version, but the messy, non-linear, sometimes-going-backward reality of a person genuinely attempting to stop betraying herself.

To every woman who shared her story with enough honesty to make these pages honest in return: this book is yours as much as mine. The reflections that land most precisely are the ones built from what you were willing to say out loud.

To the researchers, clinicians, and theorists whose work forms the scaffolding beneath these pages — Bessel van der Kolk, whose documentation of the body's relationship to unprocessed experience changed the conversation about trauma in ways that ripple through every chapter here. Gabor Maté, whose insistence on asking what happened to you rather than what is wrong with you reoriented an entire field and a significant portion of my understanding. Peter Levine, whose somatic experiencing work gave language to what bodies hold when minds refuse. John Bowlby and Mary Ainsworth, whose attachment research produced the most practically useful map of why we return to what we know even when what we know is hurting us. Judith Herman, whose work on trauma and recovery remains indispensable. Kristin Neff, whose research on self-compassion provided the scientific foundation for what this book is asking women to practice.

To the writers who came before and made this kind of directness possible — who wrote honestly about the interior lives of women without softening what they found there, who refused the tidy resolution and insisted on the complex truth, who demonstrated through their own work that the unflinching examination of difficult experience could be both artistically rigorous and genuinely useful to the people who encountered it.

To the therapists who do this work daily — who sit with people in the middle of their most difficult reckonings and hold the space with the specific combination of professional knowledge and genuine human care that the work requires. The good therapy that reaches people before, during, and after books like this one is irreplaceable, and the people who provide it deserve more acknowledgment than they typically receive.

To anyone who picked up this book in a moment of genuine need — in the middle of a situation that was costing more than you could afford, in the aftermath of something that needed to be named before it could be addressed, in the quiet where the performance finally ran out and the honest version of your life demanded to be seen — thank you for trusting that the honest version was worth engaging rather than continuing to manage.

The work you are doing is the most important work available. Not because it is dramatic. Because it is real. And real, sustained across the ordinary days that constitute a life, changes everything.

A NOTE ON CONTINUING THE WORK

This book is a beginning. It was always only a beginning.

The 110 reflections in these pages were designed to do a specific thing: to name what has been happening below the level of the names available to you, to create the specific recognition that lands in the body before the brain has caught up, to produce the kind of clarity that makes the change feel necessary rather than optional. Whether they did that — whether they reached you in the place that needed reaching — is something only you can assess, and only time will reveal the depth of the assessment.

What comes after the book is the territory the book cannot enter. Your specific relationships, your specific history, your specific daily circumstances and the specific ways that the patterns named in these pages show up inside them. The book can name the mechanisms. Only you can do the work of addressing them in the actual texture of your actual life.

Here is what that work most reliably requires.

Sustained, honest self-examination — not the kind that loops endlessly through the same material without producing movement, but the kind directed by genuine curiosity about what is actually happening rather than what you wish were happening. Journaling, if writing is a medium that opens things for you. Meditation or contemplative practice, if stillness is where your honest knowing becomes most accessible. The specific form matters less than the consistency of the practice and the genuine quality of the inquiry.

Professional support, wherever it is possible to access. The distinction between the insight this book can provide and the relational healing that genuine therapeutic work provides is significant and worth naming plainly. Therapy — specifically the kind that is trauma-informed, body-aware, and genuinely attentive to the relational patterns this book has been addressing — provides something that no book can replicate: the lived experience of being genuinely witnessed in your difficulty by another person, and the specific healing that comes from having that experience in a relationship that is consistent, boundaried, and actually capable of holding what you bring to it.

If cost or access is a barrier, many therapists offer sliding scale fees. Online therapy platforms have expanded access significantly. Support groups — both in-person and online — organized around the specific patterns this book addresses provide community with people who understand the particular texture of this work in ways that can be genuinely sustaining. The resource you can access is more valuable than the resource you cannot, and imperfect support that is actually present is more valuable than perfect support that remains theoretical.

The people in your life who are genuinely safe — who can receive the honest version of your experience without requiring you to manage their response to it, who have demonstrated through their behavior that your self-disclosure will be held with care rather than used as information against you at a later date — those people are worth investing in and worth being honest with, in the gradual, boundaried way that genuine intimacy is built. Not all at once. Not before the trust has been demonstrated. But over time, as the evidence accumulates that a specific person can hold what you offer them.

Your own body — the direct physical experience of the patterns this book has described, which the body holds with a specificity and an accuracy that the mind cannot always access. Somatic practices — yoga, body-based therapy, breathwork, movement, the specific practices that bring conscious attention to the physical dimension of what has been discussed here — provide access to material that the cognitive approaches alone cannot reach. What the body holds requires the body's participation in the releasing of it.

The writing — not necessarily formal journaling, though that is valuable for many people. The specific act of putting words to the experiences that have been lived in silence. Letters to people that will not be sent. Records of what is actually happening rather than what the performance requires. The private, honest, completely uncensored account of what your interior life actually looks like on ordinary days.

And patience — the specific, continuous, not-romanticized patience of someone who is building something that takes time. The healing from significant, sustained self-betrayal is not a project that completes on a timeline that feels adequate to the urgency of the need. It moves at the pace of genuine change, which is slower than insight and faster than giving up and entirely its own regardless of what the comparison to other people's timelines suggests.

Stay in it. Not the suffering — you are done with that loyalty. In the work. The daily, imperfect, genuinely transformative work of becoming someone who no longer organizes her life around her own pain.

That person is already in you. These pages have been working to clear the ground for her.

Now you go find her.

She has been there all along.

***

If this book reached you, consider that someone in your life may be exactly where you were when you found it. Pass it on when it feels right. The work multiplies through honest conversation and through the courage of one person willing to say to another: I found something that named what I could not name, and I thought of you.

"She did not stop suffering because the pain disappeared. She stopped because she finally refused to be the one who kept it alive."

www.ingramcontent.com/pod-product-compliance
Lightning Source LLC
LaVergne TN
LVHW022222200926
848481LV00006B/2073

* 9 7 8 9 9 9 0 9 0 5 5 1 9 *